When Alzheimer's Hits Home

Jo Danna

Palomino Press • New York

WHEN ALZHEIMER'S HITS HOME
by Jo Danna, Ph.D.

Published by:

Palomino Press
86-07 144th Street
Briarwood, NY 11435-3119 U.S.A.
(718) 297-5053

Printed and bound in the United States of America.

Publisher's Cataloging in Publication Data
Danna, Jo.
When Alzheimer's Hits Home / Jo Danna
p. cm.
Includes index.
Preassigned LCCN: 94-65719.
ISBN 0-9610036-4-2
1. D'Anna, Lucia M.--Health. 2. Alzheimer's disease--Patients--Biography. 3. Alzheimer's disease--Patients--Family relationships. 4. Alzheimer's disease--Patients--Long-term care. I. Title.

RC523.D364 1990 362.1'96831'0092
QBI94-1286

$14.95 Softcover

ACKNOWLEDGEMENTS

This book owes much to the many compassionate professionals — social workers, nursing home administrator, nurse's aides, elder law attorney — who work with Alzheimer's victims and their families. They kept the author's faith alive in moments when it was flagging. This book would not exist without them.

Special thanks also to my dear friend and colleague, Göran "George" Moberg, director of The Writing Consultant Press, and my brother, Carl Danna, retired English teacher and current actor-poet-playwrite. They offered comfort when help was needed most, and their suggestions as editors made this story more than a maudlin wallow in self-pity.

Book cover by Susan Danna

ABOUT THE AUTHOR

Jo Danna is the author of six highly acclaimed books. *When Alzheimer's Hits Home* is based on a diary she kept while taking care of her mother, an Alzheimer's victim. In this book she shares her mistakes and triumphs so others who are in a similar situation may find solace and peace and gateways to assistance.

She is a psychologist, anthropologist and educator who has been listed in several Who's Who directories: *Who's Who in America, Who's Who in American Women, Community Leaders of America, World's Who's Who of Women*. Her Ph.D. and M.A. were earned at Columbia University and her B.A. at Hunter College of the City University of New York.

CONTENTS

APPENDIX A

CAREGIVER, TAKE GOOD CARE OF YOURSELF

APPENDIX B

WHAT YOU DON'T KNOW ABOUT ALZHEIMER'S CAN HURT YOU

APPENDIX C

HELP FOR CAREGIVERS

APPENDIX D

LEGAL AND FINANCIAL INFORMATION

APPENDIX E

FOR MORE INFORMATION

LA SOFFERENZA

Years ago, when I was doing anthropological fieldwork in a Sicilian mountain village, "La Sofferenza" — the ability to triumph over great suffering — was highly valued. It was seen as a rite of initiation to prepare us for future hardships, a crucible of fire to strengthen character and put "steel" into our backbone. But there are limits. Caring for a family member who suffers from dementia is a crucible of fire no one should endure without help.

This is a story of how I and my mother, Lucy (Lucia Macaluso D'Anna) stumbled through the various stages of Alzheimer's disease. I started it to help me understand her increasingly strange behavior. Then I realized that sharing my experience with other caregivers may help them avoid some of my trials and errors in learning to manage this terrible affliction.

If you are facing a similar tragedy, I hope this book will remind you that in moments when you feel you're about to lose control, there are many people who'll want to help you. At the very least, you'll receive comfort in knowing you're not alone.

Perhaps you are too close to the problem to see how your efforts influence the sick person. You'll read how some of my caring techniques only made my mother's behavior worse and how this, in turn, increased my own frustration and anger.

Some solutions that I discovered by trial and error will lighten your burden and make the sick person more comfortable and less anxious. You may even think of better ways to resolve the unexpected dilemmas that pop up daily.

It won't be easy. There will be moments when you're about to lose control. The strain of living with and caring for a dementia victim can be so great that something eventually will snap.

I hope that reading what happened to me will inspire you to take better care of yourself. As caregivers, we become so depressed and tired that we neglect ourselves. In desperate moments, we may even struggle against the instinct to save ourselves. Don't let this happen to you! Get help early! Who will take care of the sick person if you become incapacitated or are out of the scene? Think about other members of your family.

On the other hand, the instinct for self-preservation is so strong in some caregivers, they react by hurting the sick person, as caricatured in the comedy, *Throw Mamma From the Train*. Social workers in elder care centers say that elder abuse is an ugly and growing reality. The important thing to understand is that, in the absence or shortage of affordable help for families, they do not blame the abusers.

"Dementia" is a medical term for several types of brain disorder which affect memory, personality, judgement, language, perception, and motor coordination. About 50% of dementia cases are due to Alzheimer's disease; 20% are due to multi-infarct disease (caused by small strokes in the brain); 20% come from a combination of AD and multi-infarct disease; and about 10% from other illnesses.

THE LOST SELF

Don't get me wrong. I'm not the one who has Alzheimer's Disease. My mother does. But I'm also the victim of this dreaded illness. You see, I'm her caregiver.

After a three-year teaching stint in Australia, I was looking forward to coming home. Home is Briarwood in Queens, New York City where I've lived, on and off, for years with Mom. I was expecting to resume the same relatively hassle-free, mother-daughter relationship we've always had. Instead, the relationship had changed into one of suspicion and anger, shouting and insults, often over trivial matters.

At the time I didn't know the subtle changes in her personality were early signs of a disease that was slowly destroying her mind and twisting her personality into that of a stranger. She was losing her self, the person I knew and loved.

This loss of self can also happen to a family caregiver. Like the Al-Anon member whose entire life revolves around the alcoholic, our lives are restricted by the Alzheimer victim, and we both lose a sense of who we had been. Each day is filled with crises, and every hour is focused on the sick person's needs and behavior. Gradually, we lose a sense of control over our lives. The devastation the disease wreaks on the sick person also takes its toll on us, and we become its secondary victims.

> *A change in personality is an early symptom. A trait may become exaggerated: a formerly quick tempered person now flies into fiery rages. Or it may be reversed: an energetic person becomes apathetic or a cheerful person becomes morose.*

FLASHBACK 1918

La Miseria

In a small Sicilian village perched on a pinnacle of the Madonie Mountains, so high up that flies stagger about in the dry, thin air, Lucia lay shivering from fever. "La Miseria," as the villagers called the deadly influenza virus, took millions of lives throughout Europe that year. But Lucia was young and, as she liked to brag years later, "strong enough to lift a calf." It was probably this, and the rarified atmosphere that had exhausted even this killer virus, which saved her.

So Lucia lived, but the virus left her deaf in one ear. This started the sequence of events leading to her arrival in the United States and ended with her gradual descent into madness.

In a village known for its beauties, Lucia was considered quite a catch. What's more, she could read and write. A healthy, attractive girl who worked hard in the house and vineyards and was also literate would be an asset to any young farmer. In those days rural schooling was not compulsory. For girls especially, it was considered a waste. In Lucia's case, however, the village elders would shake their heads sadly and say, "What a pity Lucia cannot continue her schooling."

It was because of the flu epidemic that she married the "rich American" instead of Armando, a lad from a neighboring village. In those days a young man courted his beloved by singing love songs under her balcony while the other villagers were supposed to be asleep. But when the sounds of mandolin music penetrated the crisp midnight air, everyone's eyes and ears were glued to their windows.

It so happened that on the night Armando came courting, Lucia was sleeping on her one good ear and she didn't hear a note. From then on, whenever they passed each other on the road, Armando would stare straight ahead as if he had not seen her. This left the field open for Domenico D'Anna.

The horror of Alzheimer's disease is the way it erases an entire existence, just as a vicious hand wipes away a life history outlined on a blackboard, leaving only shadowy traces. A person may have written a popular song, won a Nobel Prize, or raised children who later became good citizens. That person may have been a teacher who changed lives, a ballet dancer who brought joy to people, a lover. What's left is a stranger whose entire existence is diminished to a diagnostic label — *Alzheimer's victim*.

I started this diary to keep from losing my Self. I also thought it would help me understand my mother's increasingly odd behavior. At one moment Mom would be a Dr. Jekyll, her normal generous, loving and trusting self. At the next moment she'd be a hostile, suspicious, sarcastic Ms. Hyde. Better to spill out my anger and confused feelings in writing, I thought, than to scold, preach, and shout to little effect. Since keeping a diary is very much like going to confession or talking to a psychotherapist, I figured it would help.

Then, as I reviewed the events in my diary over the months and years, I noticed that my patient explanations, cajoling and, finally, angry threats made no difference in Mom's behavior. She was becoming more forgetful, more irrational, and more hostile. The diary helped me realize that she wasn't just getting ornery and stubborn in her old age. She was sick!

EARLY SIGNS OF MADNESS

It was hard to tell, really, when my brother and I felt that first stab of fear — Was Mom's mind starting to go? She was so clever at hiding the symptoms from us, maybe even to herself.

Years before the signs became too obvious to ignore, she started doing mental exercises. I remember thinking it was strange because she had never done them before; at least, not with such vengeance. In retrospect, it was as though she was trying to strengthen her waning mental powers. She would add long shopping lists mentally, refusing our offer of a pencil or calculator, and she'd read aloud from newspapers and magazines. Did all this effort prevent Alzheimer's? No, it did not. Did it help postpone the symptoms? Possibly, but who knows?

The odd incidents over the years seemed so minor no one took notice of them at the time. No one realized they were signs of a gradual disintegration of Mom's personality, the onset of Alzheimer's disease. She was once the kindest and gentlest of persons, with an open, generous nature. By the mid-1980s she was paranoid and disagreeable.

The changes are so subtle, you may not notice them in the early stage of Alzheimer's disease.

Ordinary acts like helping her prepare meals and take a bath, and reminding her it was time to go to bed had turned into epic battles. At the time, I didn't know this is typical in the early stages of dementia, and I reacted by arguing with her and yelling. "I hate you," I would sometimes say, and in my heart I wanted to murder her.

Mom Thinks I'm a Thief: Summer 1984

One day, she asked me to take her to the bank to close out her savings account. When we got home, she hid the large check and later forgot where she had put it. She accused *me* of stealing it! Soon after that incident, she started hiding her pocketbook. In our family, we always lived together in mutual trust and we never had to hide things from one another.

The Missing Gifts: Christmas 1984

She always enjoyed selecting Christmas gifts that would please each of us, but for the last few years she couldn't be bothered.

At least, that's what she said. This was another subtle change we hardly noticed.

Christmas Eve came, and her children and grandchildren gathered at our house to exchange gifts. When it was Mom's turn, the money envelopes for her grandchildren were missing. In front of everyone, she accused *me* of stealing them! Everyone's eyes were on me, filled with bewilderment and suspicion. It's hard to describe the pain of believing your family suspects you are stealing from your own mother. Since Mom seemed normal in every other respect, no one suspected this change in her personality was an early sign of Alzheimer's disease.

Mom denies the growing fear that something is wrong with her mind by blaming others for the consequences of her forgetfulness and by resisting offers of help. Later, when the disability becomes obvious even to her, she will ask for it.

The following year, as I was getting the Christmas trimmings down from the attic, I found the envelopes with the ten dollar bills. She had forgotten she had hidden them in a Santa music box.

The Man Who Loved to Buy Cadillacs

There was an old man who loved to shop in the mall. Although he was in an early stage of Alzheimer's disease, his family didn't suspect anything was wrong until the wild shopping sprees began. With his credit card he would charge television sets, refrigerators, and other expensive items. Then he'd come home relaxed and happy. The next day, having forgotten what he had bought the previous day, he would return to the mall and start all over. Once he even charged a new Cadillac. Meanwhile, back home, trucks arrived regularly to deliver television sets, refrigerators, etc. which, of course, had to be returned. Finally, after an electronics store refused a return on a fifth television set, the family had his Visa card canceled.

Mom Has Problems With Money: 1985

In retrospect, what should have alerted us was the size of Mom's change purse. It got larger and larger over the years. She was always good at mental arithmetic, but lately she had difficulty making change. She would hand the supermarket clerks big bills, and stuff the change in her pocketbook without counting it.

Alzheimer's disease is a progressive disorder which affects several areas of the brain, resulting in a variety of symptoms, the earliest and most noticeable of which are a personality change and a loss of recent memory significant enough to interfere with normal living. As the disease spreads, remote memory, abstract thinking, judgement, language ability and motor coordination are also impaired.

Mom also began having problems balancing her checkbook. When her son, Carl, scolded her for not keeping her records straight, Mom would cry. Finally, one day, he took her to the bank to cancel her checking account. She was humiliated, and Carl was riddled with guilt. Still, we would not allow ourselves to admit this was a symptom of early dementia.

"Oh, she's just getting senile. It's to be expected at her age," everyone agreed. Yet, even when the incidents became more frequent, like when our favorite supermarket clerk hinted that mom was having "a little trouble" counting her change we could not admit the obvious.

Mom Loses Her Sense of Shame: 1986

After Mom had surgery for a broken hip, she stayed with Carl near New Orleans for several months. At first, her sense of modesty and shame was still intact. Carl would scrub her back, shampoo her hair and rinse her with the shower arm, and all the while she would never expose her front. A year later, during another visit to him, Mom had lost all sense of modesty. She allowed him to bathe her naked body, front and back.

The Chinese Restaurant: 1987

The other day, something happened which reinforced my growing fears about Mom's mind. I took her for an annual checkup to the only doctor she allows to touch her naked body. He's a well-known surgeon who was born in a Mennonite community and now has a Park Avenue practice. Mom loves this six-foot redhead like a son, and he has a special affection for her. It's not so strange considering that both come from a rural farming background.

> *Just as Mom denies the growing fear that something may be wrong with her mind, members of the family deny the horror of what the subconscious mind already knows.*

On the way home, we stopped for lunch in a Chinese restaurant just off Lexington Avenue and 53rd. It's the sort of place with tables so close together that you can hear what diners at nearby tables are saying. As I leaned back to relax and watch Mom enjoy her beef and broccoli, I noticed people at nearby tables staring at us. Mom had poured tea onto her plate of rice, beef and broccoli. Then she added the won ton soup and, with a teaspoon, blended everything into an ugly, gray mush. Next, she topped the mess with crumbled fortune cookies. I kicked her lightly under the table.

"Mom, what are you doing? You're not supposed to do that!" I hissed.

FLASHBACK 1929

Mom Sails to New York City

She had never traveled alone beyond her hamlet, not even to go to church on nearby Via Nazionale. She had never seen the ocean or tasted fish until, at age nineteen, she accompanied her father to Cefalú, by the Mediterranean Sea.

Yet, as a young bride she sailed off on an ocean liner "sola" (alone). For the first time, she was leaving her family to live with a husband she hardly knew who was waiting for her in New York City. She was leaving her hamlet, which had no more than thirty residents and no electricity or plumbing, to live in the most cosmopolitan and densely populated city in the world. Imagine! There were more people on that ocean liner than in all of Gioiotti! After the ship glided past the Statue of Liberty and docked in New York harbor, there were no close relatives to greet her; there was only her brand new husband, a stranger, really.

Mom was again "sola" when her first child was delivered nine months later in a Manhattan tenement by a "stranger," a Neapolitan midwife, herself a recent immigrant. In Petralia, the rites of passage — birth, graduation, marriage, emigration, death — are celebrated by the extended family and often by the entire village. Mom "celebrated" her trip across the Atlantic Ocean and the birth of her first child "sola!" A woman with less courage might not have survived this with her sanity intact, despite the love of a "rich" husband and the excitement of living in a city where one could buy fish any time of the day or night.

"Dear Mother of God, show me how to do this!" she cried while struggling to swaddle her baby. It was squirming so vigorously that it was in danger of slipping off the kitchen table. She had often assisted mothers as a child, but this was the first time she was doing it alone, with no one to advise her. Suddenly, the Virgin Mary appeared and gently showed the young immigrant how to swaddle her first born. Mom awoke from this nightmare to find that she had swaddled her baby perfectly. The Virgin had responded to her cry for help.

"Don' tell me how I should eat!" she shouted. Her hearing was getting worse.

"Ma, people are looking at you!"

"Let them look," she replied as she chewed the mess with obvious relish. (Mom was always right.) "Everything taste good when it's in the stomach," she replied with her crazy logic.

Looking back, I see that we, her children and grandchildren, were in denial. We could accept any other medical catastrophe happening to her — a heart attack, cancer, a stroke — but not dementia. Not Mom, who had always been such strong and dominant personality that we nicknamed her *Mussolini*, and our habit of deferring to her persisted well into our adult years.

Recent memory goes first, followed by a gradual loss of distant memory. At first, Mom complained of not remembering names as well as she used to. Then, she'd forget major events of the past week. This was followed by forgetting something she had just read or seen on TV. Later still, she'd get lost coming home from shopping. Finally, she didn't recognize her house, forgot the names of her loved ones, couldn't remember where the toilet was, and that she had been married and raised three children.

HOW I MET MORRIS

Summer 1988

After spending the winter holiday in El Paso, where she drove her other daughter, Libby, crazy by always crying she wanted to "go home," Mom *is home*, but she doesn't know it.

To all outward appearances, Mom looks, talks and behaves like a normal person, at least for the first twenty minutes or so. She knows I'm her daughter, Jo. She knows her address, telephone number, birth date, the name of our President, and she recognizes her grandchildren and common food staples. She's also healthy, and can walk a mile with little difficulty. But she will suddenly announce that she's "going home" or she's going to take a walk to visit her brothers and sisters. They live in Italy.

Most healthy old people do well on tests of mental ability, and many have brain functions like that of a younger person. Any negative changes are the exception, not the rule. The culprit is illness. In one study, for example, 15% to 20% of the elderly persons tested showed no detectable changes in memory or reasoning ability. Many who did less well on the tests had something else wrong with them, such as depression, amnesia or Alzheimer's disease.

Mom walks briskly with me to the supermarket, singing "*Ce la luna mezzo mare, mamma mia voglio maritare*" ("There's a full moon over the ocean. Mamma, I want to get married.") Thinking she's "going home," she taps her cane to the happy beat all the way, stopping to smile at children who are shorter than she is, which limits this population to people under the age of nine.

She's wearing a sky blue dress that almost reaches to her ankles, and she walks with a cute toddler walk. Her face has an ecstatic expression as she holds an ice cream cone with the cream dripping down her chin. People passing by beam back the same "Oh, how adorable" type of smile that our little dog, Muffin, used to elicit when she was a puppy.

A short, good-looking man, perhaps in his early seventies, bows and doffs his hat at Mom just as they do in silent films. I've seen him occasionally on my way to the supermarket, but we've never spoken.

"Hello, my name is Morris. It's a pleasant day, isn't it?" Still bowing, he turns his gaze toward me and asks, "This is your mother?"

"Yes. Have a pleasant day," I reply impatiently.

"You live alone with your sweet mother?" he asks, his eyes fixed on the bare third finger of my left hand.

"Yes."

"In the neighborhood?"

"Not too far."

"I still work, you know. I own a factory. We make garter belts. I enjoy going to the movies and I love to dance. Do you dance?"

"It's nice meeting you. We have to rush. We're moving upstate soon," I lie.

He looks hurt, and I feel bad about brushing him off so rudely. The sweet old man is lonely, perhaps a recent widower.

Older people need what all people need to remain in optimal (mental and physical) health: work to do, money to live on, a place to live in, and other people to care whether they live or die. In fact, work is seen as probably the biggest preservative of all.
House Select Committee on Aging, August 1977

In this neighborhood there are lots of lonely old people, many of them living alone. Usually, they congregate in the bagel and coffee shop or the one-room branch library where they disturb readers with their loud talking. Most of the women put on too much makeup. They wear bouffant platinum blond wigs and clothes that are gaudy, too short and youthful. They look pathetic, not like the sexy bombshells they hope to resemble.

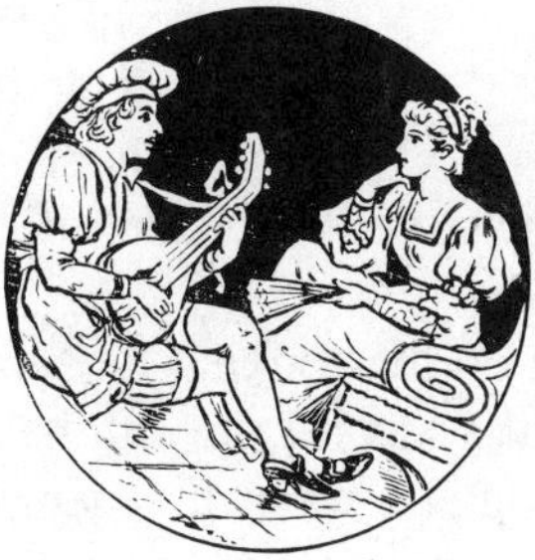

BURNT LAMB CHOPS

An Early Winter Day: 1988

Gradually, almost imperceptibly, Mom is becoming careless and slovenly. Often she's resentful of me. This is more noticeable when I'm in *her* kitchen, preparing meals *she* should be preparing. After she twice set the kitchen on fire by leaving pots on the burners and walking away, I decided to do the cooking and be present whenever she used the stove.

Ability to complete complex tasks declines gradually from the early to moderate stages. At first, the sick person may complain more than usual about his/her job. This is followed by poor work performance which co-workers start to notice, although the person is still able to do undemanding personal or job related tasks. Then, routine complex tasks such as planning and preparing dinner, handling finances, marketing, etc. become increasingly difficult. At this point the person is no longer able to perform on the job.

One evening, her granddaughter Susan came to dinner. As I started to prepare the lamb chops for broiling, Mom followed close on my heels. From her rapid, heavy breathing, I could sense she was seething with anger, but it was hard to know for sure because she usually keeps her negative feelings to herself.

"Why are you looking at me like that?"

"Nothin'!" she replied with a glare. She edged closer and closer to the stove until I could feel her hot breath on my neck.

"Okay! Okay! You do the cooking for Susan!"

This was too much! I was fed up with her hostile attitude toward me lately, as though I were the enemy. I decided to stop shielding her from her mistakes to teach her a lesson. Maybe after tonight's disaster, she'll accept my help without giving me dirty looks. The thought that she might have Alzheimer's was still too horrible to admit.

Susan and I watched Mom prepare dinner from the dining room. Mom hesitantly took the unwashed lamb chops, which had about an inch of fat around, from the wrapper and put them right on the oven grill. I had to restrain myself from telling her to put them in a pan. Susan didn't interfere either except to light the oven at Mom's request.

> *Her world has become a strange and frightening place. The mental compass which helped her navigate through her todays and tomorrows has been erased by her inability to remember familiar surroundings, objects, and loved ones. Typical reactions to this loss are denial, anger, fear, grief and depression.*

We watched in amazement as Mom scattered whole unwashed potatoes and unpeeled onions around the lamb chops. She performed each action tentatively, as if trying to recall which step comes next. The look of happiness on her face made me feel ashamed of myself.

Then we all went into the living room to catch up on family news. A delicious, pungent smell of broiling lamb chops began to fill the rooms. Mom was obviously pleased by our expressions of anticipation. Soon, there were hints of burning meat. When wisps of smoke started to swirl about the ceiling, Susan and I pretended not to notice. Soon a black cloud of grease overwhelmed the wisps of smoke. For a few moments, Susan and I pretended to chat nonchalantly. Mom tried to hide her nervousness behind a facade of dignity. Finally, panic set in. Susan and I rushed into the kitchen.

We turned off the oven, opened the door and windows, and turned on the exhaust fan. Black grease covered the walls, and lumps of charcoal had replaced the lamb chops and vegetables.

FLASHBACK 1930's

Mom "Loins" English

I'm going crazy. She has been singing, full blast, the same damn song all morning, pausing now and then to ask herself, "Where this toon came from? Who loined me this toon?"

It's a sparkling Indian summer day and I want her out of the house, "Ma, why don't you take a nice walk?"

"I like to go but my legs and back doesn't budget"

Years ago, while we were in elementary school, Mom taught herself to speak and read English. She used to wait outside, with a newspaper in hand, for me to come home from school. Suddenly, she would collar me or one of my friends and ask, "How you say this woid?" "What this woid means?"

To this day, her fractured English and spelling is the delight of everyone and proof that she's self- taught. What difference did it make since she could read the newspaper, soup can labels, bills, and letters from her children?

- *For "usually," "as a rule," or "generally," she would say, "General, as a ruler ...."*
- *Customers in the bakery shop would wonder, then titter, as Mom ordered "holy wheat bread" and "half dozen fresh beagles, please."*
- *I often made her "go bear sick." (bezerk)*
- *My favorites were "Don' jump outta conclusion!" and*
- *"Don' do things on the sperm of the moment!*

"Excellent! What seasonings did you put in?" Susan and I pretended to enjoy the dinner. We knew Mom had forgotten to add them.

The evening had started with my hoping shock therapy would make Mom realize her powers were declining, and she should accept my help without arguments and hostile looks. Now I hated myself for putting her through an embarrassing ordeal. She looked small and pathetic as she tried to maintain her dignity by pretending things were just fine, that the pieces of burnt meat we tried to swallow were delicious.

MOM INVITES THIEVES IN FOR LUNCH

Early Spring 1989

It was on a cool April day this year that my conscious mind finally admitted the awful truth. Increasingly, over the years there had been incidents in which she exhibited a nasty, slovenly and forgetful side that was so uncharacteristic of her. It was easier to explain these incidents away as senility, "natural" at age eighty-seven.

Although in the moderate stage, sick persons still recognize familiar persons, they begin to mistake strangers for "family." Knowledge of current and recent events is fading, and gaps in the memory of one's own personal history increase.

Dementia? Not in Mom, who had always been a paragon of common sense, who was so proud of her amazing ability to remember dates, names, and events far into the past, who always admonished us kids to "Use your logic! Don't do things on the *sperm* of the moment!" Take, for example, the harsh comments she'd now make about her neighbors and relatives. Coming from a woman who rarely made an unkind remark about anyone, it's as if a part of her personality had split into a dark side.

Even more frightening is that she now mistakes any stranger who rings the doorbell as "family." One day, about 1:30 p.m., while I was upstairs, I heard women's voices in the living room. "That's strange. Kristen is early," I thought as I ran downstairs to greet Mom's granddaughter. Instead, I saw two strangers, young women, probably in their twenties. From the neck up they seemed slender, but it was hard to tell since they wore billowing, ankle length skirts over what looked like bulging abdomens. Babushkas, those large, multi--colored scarves Russian peasant women wear over their hair, hid part of their face. They each carried two very large straw bags. They seemed very charming.

A person with Alzheimer's can live 20 years or more from the onset of symptoms.

"Come sit," Mom said as she began setting four places at the table for lunch.

"Excuse me, do I know you?" I asked politely.

In an accent I could not identify, the taller woman replied, "We were visiting our friend who lives next door, but nobody's home. I rang your doorbell because my sister here is pregnant,"she gently patted her sister's bulging stomach, "and she was almost fainting from thirst. Your mother was kind enough to let us in." The "sister" rubbed her abdomen and smiled faintly.

"Are you from Europe?" I asked.

"No, from Israel," she replied in an accent that was definitely *not* Israeli.

Nothing in their demeanor suggested nervousness or anything out of the ordinary. But my sixth sense told me something fishy was going on.

Molly, our neighbor, is a fun-loving, ninety-three year old Irish woman who walks half a mile, six days a week, to play bingo. I couldn't believe she'd be expecting two "friends" from Israel and in their twenties no less to visit during bingo time.

"What's your friend's name?" I asked.

"Shumila," the tall one replied, still smiling coolly.

"Her name is Molly! She's from Dublin, and she's ninety-three years old!" I almost shouted.

Without a trace of nervousness, she replied, "Oh, not that neighbor. Our friend lives two houses down."

"That house has been empty for three years!" I said.

By the time family members notice something is wrong, the disease may no longer be in the early stages. At first, we didn't realize Mom had Alzheimer's disease, she was so good at hiding her growing disability from us. She was still able to do most of the things she had always done, such as light shopping and housekeeping, preparing simple meals, and bathing and dressing herself.

The "pregnant" one, looking at her watch, said, "We must go. We have an appointment."

"Would you like some water before you leave?" I said, hoping to fool them into thinking that I was not going to call the police as soon as they got out the door.

The "pregnant" one hurriedly took a few sips and went out the door fast.

"You'll probably think this is not an emergency," I said to the 911 operator apologetically. I explained what happened.

"Hold on," she said, "a detective wants to speak with you."

After putting down the receiver, I yelled at Mom, "Don't you *ever* open the door to a stranger again, you hear!"

This made her furious because I had violated the Sicilian code of respect toward one's elders. "I thought it was Kristen with her friend," she said defensively.

The detective came sooner than expected. Hearing a man's voice in the living room, I ran downstairs again to find Mom smiling at a short, thin man, about fortyish. He had dark brown hair and eyes and was wearing jeans, a scruffy T-shirt, and sneakers. "Special unit," he said, showing his badge.

As a progressive disorder which affects several areas of the brain, Alzheimer's disease shows a variety of symptoms. Therefore, you cannot assume a person has AD on the basis of one or two symptoms.

He explained that a detective unit has been trying to solve a series of crimes against elderly people in Queens. The criminals are two young females who "work" daytime hours when no one else is likely to be home. They use the ruse of being pregnant and feeling faint to get inside a house where an elderly face is looking blankly out a window.

It's easy to spot a lonely old person in a big city and to evoke his/her compassion. Once inside, one criminal distracts the good Samaritan with conversation while the other ransacks the house. Earlier this year, these criminals knocked down and killed an elderly man in their rush to get out of the house after his daughter unexpectedly walked into a room they were ransacking.

Not more than ten minutes had elapsed between the time I first hollered at Mom for letting in the two strangers and the time she invited the plainclothes detective to come in. I was furious. It didn't occur to me that something was wrong with her mind. She was angry, too. "I thought it was Peter! Can't I even let in my own grandson?"

FLASHBACK 1970

"Sola" in Petralia Soprana

In Mom's day in Petralia, and to a lesser extent today, a respectable young woman was rarely seen out of doors. Nor did she venture far from the side of an older female relative if she wanted to keep her reputation "spotless."

As a young, Italian-American anthropologist doing research in Petralia, whenever I set out to do some observation or administer psychological tests, whenever I just wanted to walk alone along the cloud covered mountain road, an older female relative would rush up and grab my arm.

"Sola? (alone?) Where are you going?" the chaperon would ask, out of breath from trying to keep up with my New York pace. The dear souls were anxious to preserve my chastity.

Despite all my book learning in anthropology, I never imagined how profoundly unnerving the cultural differences could be. I had expected the villagers, my relatives especially, to understand that as an American woman I am different from them. I am "libera" (free, independent). I am an individualist. Growing up in New York City has helped me overcome the herd instinct.

The very idea of developing one's unique personality, of "doing your own thing" was difficult even for the teenagers of Petralia, the future residents of the 21st Century, to grasp! I had administered a psychological test to students at the middle school in town. One statement they were to complete was, "A person who tries to distinguish him- or herself from others is -----." Their responses were nearly unanimous: Such a person is "not to be respected!"

"SOLA" IN NEW YORK CITY

Maybe this is one reason why Mom is so eager to accompany me on shopping trips, why she sings and talks incessantly. Mom now lives like a typical urban American. Her son lives near New Orleans and another daughter in Texas. The old neighbors, first generation immigrants from Northern Europe, are gone and a new wave of immigrants have moved in. Her closest friends now are a Sri Lankan family whose children come over often to play with our poodle and a recently arrived woman from India. These persons comprise her "extended family."

Is Mom always wanting to go to church the lonely old woman's equivalent of teenagers wanting to join a gang? Each seeks a sense of "belonging." Each needs the companionship of like-minded souls to ease the pain of existing in a state of social limbo. Each wants to escape, even for a moment, the feeling of not belonging, of being discarded by the rest of society.

OUR LADY OF THE CENACLE RAPS TO A LATIN BEAT

The Following Sunday

I feel virtuous accompanying Mom to church because it's been such a long time. I'm hoping she'll see one of her old Irish, German or Scottish neighbors there. As she blesses herself with holy water at the entrance to the packed church, her eyes shine with anticipation as they search the crowd eagerly.

When the Mass begins, Mom wears the relaxed look that comes from a well-practiced ritual. As the priest starts to speak, she cranes her neck and turns her one good ear toward the altar. Soon her smile of anticipation changes to a bewildered look.

The Mass is in Spanish! We may be the only non-Hispanic persons present. It takes Mom a while to realize that changes have taken place in her beloved church. After that, I took her to a Unitarian church which is closer. It has a multi-ethnic, multi-racial congregation and a Scottish-American minister! Mom is back in her old neighborhood again.

MOM BRINGS HOME NEW NEIGHBORS

Autumn 1989

Now, every time Mom gets lost I meet neighbors I've never seen before. Today she invited home two recent immigrants from Thailand, young women who live on the next street. They had seen her tottering around on her cane, looking confused, and brought her home. Thank God, she still knows her address.

When Mom invites a stranger who brings her safely home to come inside for a cup of coffee, she sees the dignity and humanity of the person, not the foreign accent or skin color. "We're all God's creatures under the sun," she used to say when she still had her mind.

When the United Nations was founded in 1947, the Briarwood-Flushing area of Queens was its first site. Mom used to watch, fascinated, as people in saris and other exotic garb walked to the subway down the street. Even today, she views people of different color and facial pattern as the elite of their respective cultures, not as different and, therefore, to be feared or despised.

Mom's social skills were still intact in the early and middle stages of Alzheimer's disease.

The following Sunday another neighbor I had not met before, this one speaks with an Irish lilt, brought Mom home from Mass.

FLASHBACK 1969

Sunday Mass in Petralia Soprana

La Trinita Church is perched on a pinnacle of the Madonie Mountains, at the crossroads between several outlying hamlets of Petralia Soprana. Villagers, dressed in their Sunday best, are standing outside in the crisp, clear mountain air, waiting for Mass to begin.

Gathering for Sunday Mass gives them psychological benefits as well as spiritual benefits. They can think of themselves as "people of Petralia Soprana" rather than of this or that tiny hamlet. You see, the town residents have instilled an inferiority complex in their rural cousins — a sense of being ignorant, rough, and easily fooled. Attending mass also binds the extended families, many of them living in near isolation, into a single community.

It also serves as a marriage broker. While married men and women chat near the open church doors, brilliant sunlight dances in and out, and small children chase each other around the piazza. The unmarried young adults stand as far from the church as possible because they have another purpose in attending Sunday Mass.

Courtship in Petralia begins with the eyes. So, in order to get a better view of the young women who stand in tight, small groups, gossiping and giggling, the young men sit together atop the surrounding stone wall. While waiting for the signal that Mass is about to begin, a young swain looks the young beauties over to see who appeals to him most. By some sort of mysterious silent language, the chosen one understands she is being singled out. If she's interested, she returns the compliment with long, demure glances. From then on, whenever the two happen to meet — in town, at county fairs, while waiting for the bus — smoldering glances are exchanged. This can go on for months until the young man decides it's time to make his move.

He first reveals his intentions to his closest friends and then to his family. The word passes on to the girl's friends and family. Next, members of both families start making discrete inquiries into the moral character of the young man or woman, how much property the family owns, the family's reputation, health, and so on. Finally, a close relative of the young man (usually the mother) pays several visits to the girl's family. With every visit they learn more about each other and about the acceptability of the proposed union to the families involved. Deciding whom to marry is not an individualistic matter as it is in the USA.

When Mass begins, the villagers stroll casually inside where they continue their conversation even after having seated themselves. Whenever I was present, the parishioners had seated themselves as far from the altar as possible, where they could continue their gossiping with little disturbance from the sermon. This didn't seem to bother the priest.

During the Catholic Mass, a little bell signals to the worshipers when it's time to beat their chests, stand, sit or kneel. One of my enduring fears as a child attending Mass in New York was to be caught out of synchrony with other parishioners. They would be standing while I was still seated or, worst yet, I would be standing when they were on their knees. I couldn't believe my eyes at the lack of concern with synchrony in Petralia. Each parishioner did his own thing. When the bell signaled it was time for kneeling, some villagers stood while others sat without the slightest indication of embarrassment!

"Armando, why are some people still sitting when we should all be kneeling?" I asked my college educated young cousin.

"Giuseppina, it's because in Italy we do not have the freedom to choose our religion as you Americans have. Those who kneel are Catholics. Those who stand are Protestants. And those who remain sitting are Atheists," he explained.

"Zia Rosina," I ask my aunt, "Why are some people sitting or standing when they should be kneeling?"

"My child, those who are seated are tired from working in the fields since dawn. Those who kneel are not too tired, and those who stand have had a good morning's rest," she explained. It was all very logical.

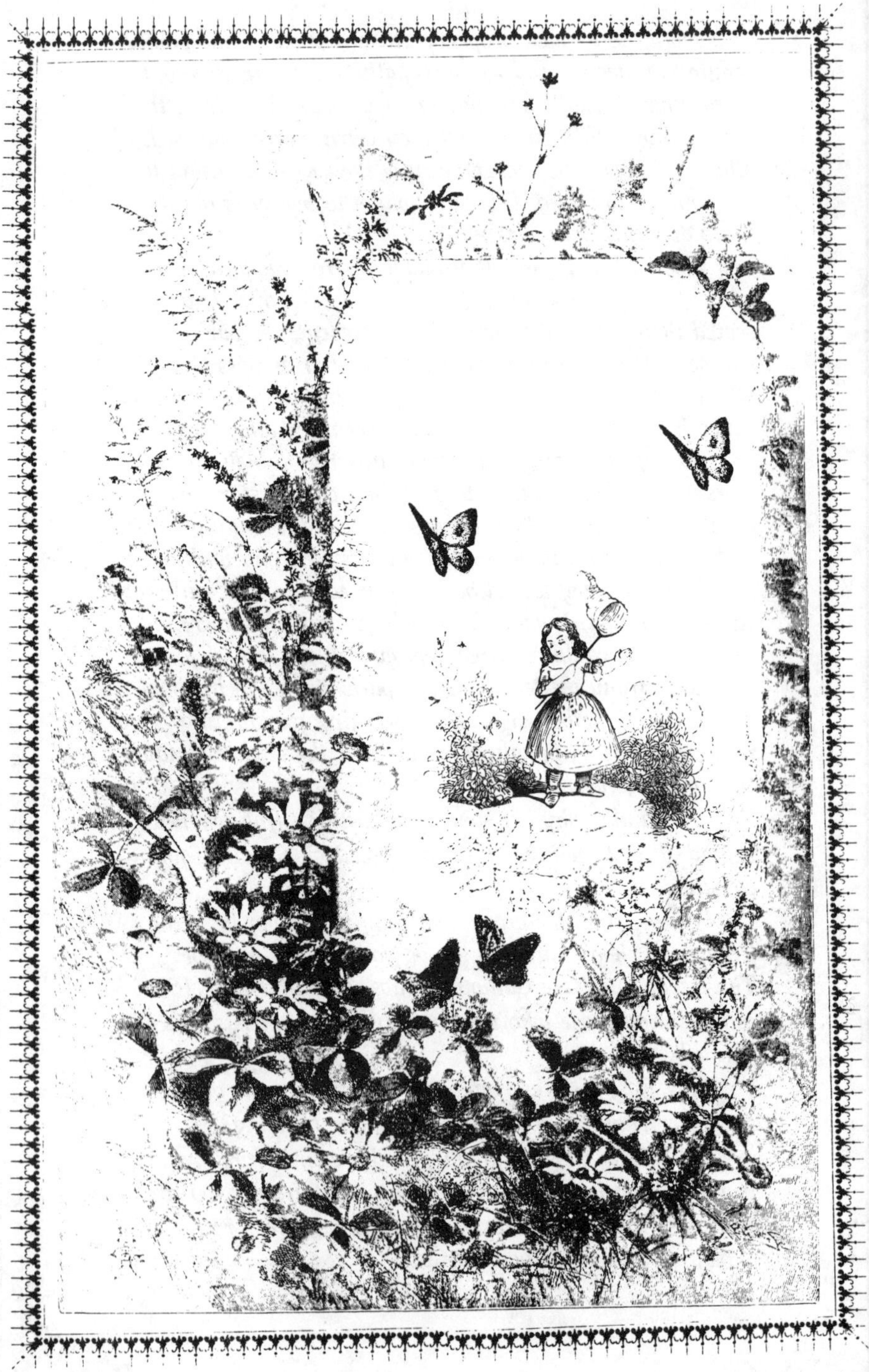

Mom had sneaked out without telling me where she was going. How she managed to walk the quarter mile and get across the expressway I'll never know. The overpass bridge has been the site of muggings recently, especially of elderly pedestrians who can be easily trapped there.

"She sat next to me in church. Since I live in this direction I brought her home," the woman said with a tone of disapproval.

Do I imagine an accusing finger pointing to my lapsed Catholic heart?

"She loves Mass so much it's a shame she has to go alone," she said in an admonishing tone. "It's dangerous."

OCEANS CHANGE, BUT NOT MOM

Mid-Summer 1990

It's a hot, humid Tuesday in Briarwood. Since 4:00 a.m. Mom has been checking into my room to see if I'm awake. She's eager to go to Sunday Mass again, although it's midweek. I pretend to be fast asleep. Then, at 5:15 a.m. she shouts, loud enough to wake the neighbors, from the bottom of the stairs,

"Jo! ***JO!*** Where are you? I'm goin' to choich!"

I bolt out of bed and rush downstairs. She hasn't even had breakfast and she's already at the front door.

On one foot she wears a dirty white sneaker and on the other a blue slipper. Over her housecoat she has on an autumn-weight dress, and around her hips a brassiere is tied like

The risk of developing Alzheimer's disease increases with very old age. At 65, the risk is about 1-2 in every 100 persons; at 80, it's 1 in 5. The good news is that even at age 80, 4 out of 5 persons do not develop the illness.

Sense of time and place is gradually lost in Alzheimer's Disease, but in the type of dementia caused by strokes or an acute physical illness, it can happen suddenly. Mom, for example, would ask, several times within minutes, what day, time or year it is. If I stepped out of sight for a few minutes, she would become agitated, and visiting people with her had become a nightmare because she would demand to go home minutes after we arrived.

a belt. Over all, she wears a winter coat. Anticipating the worst, I had already grabbed one of her summer dresses and clean underwear before rushing downstairs.

"Take off your clothes, Ma. Put these on."

She gives me an argument, as usual. Still sleepy, I have no patience to humor her.

"Put on clean underwear or you'll stink in church!" I shout.

Meekly, but reluctantly, she peels off two pairs of "bloomz," then stops.

"Take that off too!"

She objects, "I need this pair bloomz."

"Take it off!"

She does as I say, while insisting angrily that they're clean. Now I see why she didn't want to take them off in front of me. They are soiled.

"Oh, God! Did she poop in her panties?"

"I don't know how this happened" she says meekly.

Then I point to her mismatched "shoes."

"I didn't finish dressing yet," she explains, still insisting that her underwear is clean.

After I help her dress properly, she turns toward the front door again, happy and excited, expecting to see her sisters and brothers at the church.

"Ma, they live in Italy, across the ocean," I explain for the umpteenth time.

This geography lesson has been going on for more than a year. I've pointed out on a map the vast Atlantic Ocean that separates her home in New York City from Italy. I've reminded her about her first ocean trip to New York as a young bride. I've posted signs on the inner door:

> *It's impossible to walk to Italy to see your relatives. The only way is to take an airplane or swim across the ocean.*

But nothing seems to work. This is a woman whose brain used to soak up information faster than a Bounty towel soaks up coffee spills. As I again point to the spot on the map where Petralia should be, Mom shakes her head in wonderment,

"My, how things have changed!" She pauses, "I'm goin' to choich anyway."

"There's no Mass at this hour," I lie.

Her brain is like Swiss cheese. She sounds rational in bits and pieces, but there are lots of holes in her memories, especially those that process space and time relationships. For example, our house in Queens is near the top of a steep hill and, as in Petralia, there has always been a "church up the hill" but it's now a Hindu temple.

"Where's the milk?" she asks. It's right in front of her. I point to it.

"Oh, I didn't see it." She bolts down her cereal, takes a few sips of coffee and rushes toward the door again.

> *By the moderately severe stage Alzheimer victims need help in order to survive. Although they need no help with toileting and eating, they cannot take tub baths and have difficulty washing and drying themselves. Often, they don't know the date, day of week and/or season, or where they are located. They still remember their own name and the names of immediate family members, but they have forgotten other major facts about their life, such as phone number.*

What do you expect me to do, put a leash on her? Cage her up like an animal? Of course not! So I decide to risk letting her go for a walk by herself because I've got too much work to do. But first I quiz her:

"What's your address? What's your name?" She gives the correct answers. I figure that if she gets lost, at least she'll be able to tell where she lives. My morning has hardly begun and I'm already exhausted. As I close the door behind Mom, I pray that she doesn't come back, at least for a few days until I catch up on lost sleep. Also, I worry for her safety. This is how caregivers get torn apart by conflicting emotions. The stress causes physical and emotional exhaustion. Some caregivers become seriously ill from the unrelenting, severe stress. Some die!

BELLE OF THE BALL

Late Summer 1990

"Give the little lady a hand," the deejay shouts into the microphone. He's pointing to Mom, who has been dancing most of the evening at her granddaughter Laura's wedding. Earlier, Laura greeted her in the lobby of the church and mom asked, "Do I know you?"

She looks like a little granny doll in her aquamarine dress flecked with silver threads, with a silver band on her hair, and a fake diamond star pinned to her dress. (I selected the clothes.)

At four feet, eleven inches, she's the tiniest person in the hall, and she looks like a silver top twirling around and around. The young giants dancing nearby smile at her as they carefully avoid trampling on her, and she's in heaven.

After the wedding, Mom talks of the good time she had dancing.

"I gave pep to the young people. I was dancin' to give a good example. They shouldn't be afraid of gettin' old. They can enjoy life, too. You're never too old to do somethin' happy."

"Ma, do you enjoy life?"

"Certainly I enjoy life!" she always answers to my amazement.

"Ma, do you feel old?"

"I never think I'm old. I feel young." She dances a few polka steps to show her sprightliness.

CLEAN BLOOMZ

Winter 1990

In the early stages of dementia, Mom was still able to select what she'd wear for the day, dress herself properly, mail letters for me, clean her room, and wash dishes. The only time she needed help was to write checks and balance her checkbook, get in and out of the tub, and do the heavy shopping, cleaning, and cooking. Now that I'm constantly exhausted, I realize how much these so-called trivial skills meant to me, for as long as she had them.

It was this month that I first noticed she'd put on four or more underpants and wear the same underwear for three or more days. I'd find smelly, blood stained undergarments tucked neatly among the freshly laundered ones in her dresser. When I talked to her about this, she grew defensive and angry. I solved the problem by hiding her clean underwear in my room.

Alzheimer sufferers retain some ability to enjoy life even in the later stages of dementia.

It's 6:30 a.m. and she's happy, almost manic, as she dresses to go to church. She expects to see her relatives and old neighbors there.

"They're in Italy, Mom!"

She's not convinced.

Many healthy elderly people who have an active social life and lots of friends, who engage in mentally stimulating activities, maintain their mental alertness and intellectual vigor until very late old age.

"They've either died or moved away!"

Again, she's not convinced.

I give up, "Okay, put these on."

"I changed my bloomz already!" She pushes away the clean underwear I hand her.

"When?"

"This mornin'!"

"That's impossible because I hide your clean underwear. The ones you have on stink!"

"No! No! My bloomz are clean! I don't want to change them."

It seems there is no way I can get her to take off her dirty underwear short of removing them by force. The verbal tug of war continues until I'm exhausted from arguing with her, but mostly from feeling guilty about wanting to knock some sense into her.

Instead of killing myself with constant arguing, I choose a rational solution. From now on I'll put clean underwear on her dresser and allow her to change when she wants. So what if she smells bad? So what if the neighbors and grandchildren think I'm neglecting her? Do they really understand what I'm going through? Let them think what they want. Some day, God forbid, they may have to live through a similar tragedy and then they'll understand. I feel my blood pressure going down.

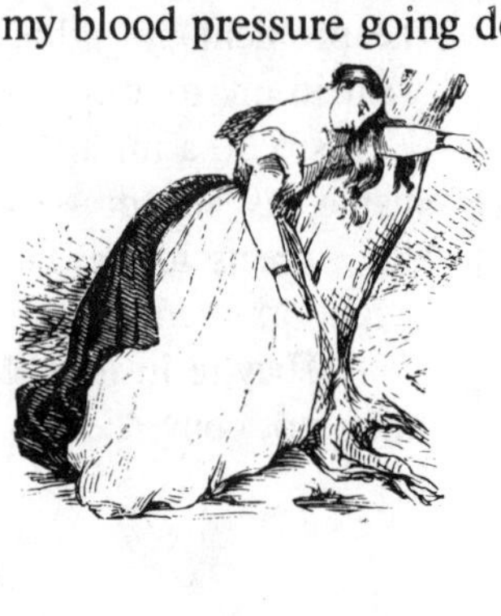

BINGO

Spring 1991

This morning she's sullen because I'm not paying attention to her. Ordinarily I make a big show of singing along with her, and listening to her talk about the same limited repertoire of topics: her children, grandchildren, poppa, grandpa, mama, the house.

I've been up since 6:45 a.m., doing chores Mom used to do for herself: selecting clothes she'd wear for the day, doing her laundry, helping her get dressed, setting out her breakfast, rubbing cream on her parched epidermis. Then she sits at the breakfast table like a lump, waiting for me to pour milk into her cereal bowl.

Delusions and hallucinations may develop in a later stage. Delusions are misinterpretations of real events or a failure to recognize loved ones. Hallucinations involve seeing, smelling, or hearing things that aren't real. The person may become dangerous at this stage if she tries to carry out what the voices are telling her to do or defend herself against imaginary threats.

I'm in a bad mood. She expects me to wait on her hand and foot, and she wants me to entertain her as well. Why doesn't she watch television or go out with Molly?

Mom's nuclear family has been her whole world in this country. She never joined clubs or accepted invitations from Molly next door to go play Bingo. Her relations with the neighbors have always been friendly but distant.

At this moment our ninety-three year old neighbor, Molly, is getting ready to go out to play Bingo. She has already done light housekeeping, washed and hung out the laundry, and gotten her three elderly male boarders settled for the day. I wish Mom had been more like Molly.

Molly's mind is alert and her memory is probably sharper than mine in my present circumstances. She walks about a half-mile a day, six days a week, to play her beloved bingo. Even when she's not feeling well, even when the weather is rotten, she won't miss her bingo. On Sundays, after cleaning the house, she usually has some of her many friends over for a game of poker. She's been doing this for fifty-five years.

MUFFIN

Early Summer 1991

Mom wants to pay me, a "nice lady," for taking care of her. She believes her son is her brother. When she's sufficiently alert to watch television, she gets upset during a violent scene, thinking it involves her family and is happening in the room.

It's a lazy summer afternoon and Mom is fantasizing again. She blends people, places and dates that bear no relation to each other into a new reality. The relationship intensifies each time she repeats the story. At first the important person smiles at Mom, then greets her, and finally speaks to her.

"I remember when I took Muffin in my arms and we went to vote in the school up the street."

It's true that the other voters probably made a fuss over the cute puppy. But gradually the presidential candidate, either George Bush or Ronald Reagan, and his wife appear in the scene. At first they appear as bystanders. Then they smile at Muffin. Finally they speak to Mom.

"Whom did you vote for, Ma?"

She's confused and doesn't answer.

"Did Muffin vote, too, Ma?" I tease.

"You make funny outta me?" she replies half jokingly.

"Of course not."

She stops short of making this final, ludicrous connection and I wouldn't be surprised if eventually she says Muffin voted too. Muffin, by the way, would have been eight years old at the time, so Mom's time frame is way off as well.

Pets have beneficial effects on mind and body. High blood pressure and chronic depression are eased, and even catatonic patients start to speak and respond. Visits to old people in nursing homes now often include bringing dogs and cats to play with.

The little poodle seems to understand that something is wrong with "Grandma." When I say, "Go kiss Grandma," she obediently goes to Mom, with head bowed, and turns back quickly before Mom has a chance to pet her. At times, when Mom sobs like a child, "What's happenin' to me? I'm nothin' any more," Muffin runs to me and I swear she has a concerned look on her sweet little face. If I don't pay attention, she paws at my knee until I get up to see what's wrong with "Grandma."

Months later, Mom began her midnight wanderings about the house, searching for her "home" and "daughter, Jo." Once she even wandered outside nearly naked. Muffin seemed to sense that Mom should be safe in bed, and she'd bark softly by my bedroom door to wake me up. Once Mom left the front door open, something you don't do if you want to survive in this city. After this incident, I slept fitfully on the front sofa until I had special locks put on all doors leading to outside.

How can anyone survive such a crisis without a pet? Muffin provides Mom and me with fun, companionship, and endless love. If not for her, I would have gone crazy by now, and Mom would be even more unbearable to live with. Now that I can't get out much, Muffin is our main source of fun and social interaction. Would two toy poodles be better than one?

THE LAYERED LOOK

A Torpid Summer Afternoon in 1991

At 4:50 p.m. I stop Mom as she's about to leave the house for "morning Mass." She's "dressed up" to meet her relatives who, she believes, are waiting for her there. She has on two dresses, one blouse and, over that, another dress. Underneath she has on two slips and three "bloomz." Over all, she wears her corset. On one foot she has a bedroom slipper. On the other foot, she had put on a stocking *over* her shoe. She looks happy, "I feel nice and warm."

From now on I decide to supervise everything she wears.

By late November, she seems to realize that she needs help in getting dressed. At times she even swallows her pride and asks for it. "I'm nothin' without you," she says softly as I help her put on a coat.

"Sexuality is part of our adulthood. It deserves to be considered. Sometimes sex becomes a problem in a dementing illness, but sometimes it remains one of the good things a couple still enjoys."

The 36-Hour Day, by Nancy Mace & Peter Rabins (Johns Hopkins University Press)

"Young" Lovers Elope

At eighty-five, our neighbor, Maria, was still attractive. Her looks meant a lot to her, and she would spend hours on her makeup and wardrobe. She had a boyfriend, Joe, a spry and alert ninety-year-old. Every day he would show up about lunch time, bow and tip his hat, and ask, "Can Maria come to lunch with me?"

The friendship became serious enough to concern Maria's family. You see, Maria was in the early stage of Alzheimer's disease, and they knew the situation would become hopeless.

Her granddaughter had a serious talk with Joe about Maria's condition, hoping to dissuade him. But he persisted, and the two "lovers" would continue to sneak out for lunch dates.

One day, Maria did not return home by late afternoon as was her custom. She was gone all night and most of the following day. Joe at first expressed ignorance of her whereabouts, but then admitted she was living in his apartment. They had eloped! For five years they lived together quite happily. He adored her and did everything he could for her. Eventually, her condition became serious enough that she had to be admitted to a nursing home, and Joe lived alone until he died.

MOM FALLS IN LOVE

A Summer Day, 1991: at Breakfast

Mom thinks the handsome, forty-five year old lawyer who administered her liability lawsuit is in love with her. Well, didn't she get his undivided attention on the day of the trial six weeks ago? And, with true love, why should a forty-five year difference matter?

Eight years earlier, when she first consulted with Mr. M., she was able to describe in detail how the bus door closed abruptly causing a hip fracture. A year later, at the deposition, she again presented the facts accurately. She understood Mr. M's professional function and she kept track of important dates, including the number of days until the trial.

> *Often what people miss most is not the act of sexual intercourse, but the touching, holding, and affection that exist between two people.*
>
> *The 36-Hour Day, by Nancy Mace & Peter Rabins (Johns Hopkins University Press)*

Since that day in a Texas courtroom, she has spoken of him

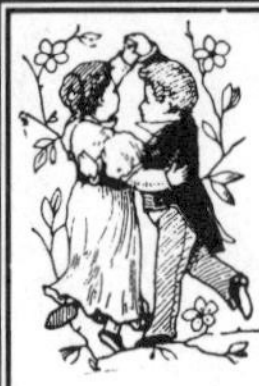

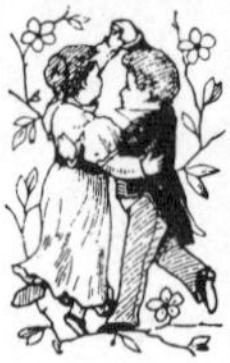

FLASHBACK 1970

Dancing in Gioiotti

Mom's version of the "denz" (the jury trial) is relevant to the hamlet in Petralia she left over sixty years ago. There are some similarities to a dance in a dimly lit barn I attended there years ago.

In Texas, twelve jury members, a judge and several observers looked on as the young lawyer lavished attention on her. This "proves" he has fallen in love with her. Nothing I say can convince her otherwise.

In Gioiotti, chairs were lined up against the barn walls facing the sawdust-covered dance floor so the "jury" and "courtroom observers" could watch the "proceedings" while a band played Sicilian country music on mandolins and guitars. (Mom has apparently overlooked this dissonant element.) Like crows huddled together on a clothesline, solemn-faced mothers, aunts, and whiskered old nonne (grannies) — most dressed in black — watched the young couples who were dancing. Apparently, to Mom's ancient eyes, these women represented the jury and courtroom observers who looked on as Mom and the lawyer danced a ritual "courtship dance."

As I chattered with my handsome young cousin on the dance floor, I noticed the other couples weren't smiling or laughing, nor were they exchanging words. They were even avoiding each other's eyes.

"Emilio, why aren't these couples talking or smiling?"

"Giuseppina," he explained, "it is not the custom in these parts to talk or laugh with your partner while dancing."

"But what's wrong with talking? And why are these old women sitting around watching with hawk eyes as the young people dance?"

At first he wouldn't answer. later I learned it was to prevent "arrangements" to meet in a hay loft later.

often, but not as her lawyer, because she has completely forgotten the accident and the attendant legal process.

"Mr. M., he took me to a denz."

"Dance? How do you know it was a dance?"

"A lotta people was sittin' around. He sat with me all evening. You think Mr. M., he liked me?"

"Yes, Ma," I lie.

She takes a sip of coffee. "You think he fell in love with me?"

"Ma, you're ninety and he's forty-two years old!"

"Age means nothin'" she says with confidence.

"Ma, he's married with two children!" I lie.

She continues eating her Cheerios, but with exaggerated non-chalance, trying to hide her disappointment. Now, three weeks later, she's still haunting me about Mr. M. She uses the pretext of calling Libby, her other daughter in Texas, daily to get more news about him.

"You think Mr. M., he will be there?"

"No, Ma, he's a very busy lawyer."

A few hours later: "I'm gonna take a walk to see Libby and maybe Mr. M, he will be there too."

Two Months Later, at Breakfast

"Could be that Mr. M. falls in love with an older lady?"

This question comes like a bolt of lightning. She has not mentioned his name in weeks, and I had assumed that her memory of him was fading, but it's still there, submerged somewhere.

"You think Mr. M. would've asked me to marry him if Libby didn't interfere?"

MOM'S SLOWLY VANISHING SELF

An Indian Summer Day 1991

Most people find it hard to understand the devastating impact dementia has on someone who, for the first ten minutes or so, looks and acts like the same person they've always known. In Mom the deterioration becomes more rapid and noticeable as the weeks go by.

It's early evening and Mom is singing like a bird. She expects her granddaughter to drop by for dinner. Earlier, I had placed two dresses on her bed to fool her into thinking she has a choice. She appears at lunch wearing one dress. Afterwards, she excuses herself. Several minutes later she reappears in the other dress. Later again, she comes in wearing a dress I had hidden in the back of her closet.

I race into her room and see that my worst fears are realized. Every piece of clothing in her closet is scattered about the room. I'm on the verge of tears.

"Ma, why did you change? You looked so good with the first dress you had on."

"Well, I had to get dressed for Kristen."

"But you *were* dressed up!"

"I was?" she answers in surprise.

Mornings after breakfast are peaceful. But as daylight fades, Alzheimer victims become restless and more confused. Mom makes little bundles and leaves them lying about the house. She paces up and down, wanting to "go home." It drove me nuts, and I'd lash out at her, but that only made things worse. Finally, after learning that this behavior, called sundowning, is due to brain damage, I was better able to tolerate it.

Next Day, At Breakfast

She remembers the president is "Mr. Bush" and his wife is "Barbara." She remembers how they met when they were young. "She came from a rich family. He was a good lookin' man." But she doesn't recognize the milk or the box of cereal.

She wants to visit her other daughter in Texas. I explain that Libby has no time or room for room for her, but she insists that Libby "needs" her.

"That's okay; I can walk there by myself."

"Ma, you can't walk from New York City to El Paso; it's too far away. You have to take an airplane. It costs one thousand dollars," I lie.

This shuts her up, but only momentarily. She repeats the refrain all day and throughout the week, and announces her imminent departure for El Paso as though for the first time, each time. I feel like running away.

It helps to understand the terror of slowly losing your memory and mental abilities by imagining yourself in the sick person's condition.

She wonders why her son (who lives on the Gulf Coast) hasn't come to visit her.

"Carl probably went to see Janice in Petralia." (Janice, her son's married daughter, lives in Long Island, New York, U.S.A.!)

"Do you know anyone in Petralia, Mom?"

"I don't remember."

Minutes Later

It's a bright, cool morning. Frank Sinatra is crooning on the radio and Mom is happy.

"I feel like goin' to Petralia! I'm goin' to see my mother." — pause — "My mother, she's dead? Oh, I forgot, she's dead," she sobs. "My father, he's still alive?" — Sob! She cries at length.

Five-thirty, Next Morning

She's already dressed to "walk" to El Paso again. She puts on the light in my room.

"Go to bed, dammit!" I shout.

She returns to her room.

One Month Later

Much of the time, she doesn't know who I am, and rarely speaks of her son or of Poppa. It's always about her daughter Libby.

"Where's Libby? She didn't say goodby to me before she left this mornin'."

Still Later

"Libby bought that tree." She's looking at some fichus tree I gave her as a gift a few months ago for the living room.

"No, Ma, I bought it."

Two Minutes Later

"That's from Libby."

Five Minutes Later

"Will you walk with me to Libby's? Why doesn't she come over?"

The holes in her memory are growing bigger and more numerous; whatever I say to her rushes right through. I'm exhausted from explaining why it's impossible to walk to Texas. Later I tell her, "This afternoon, after lunch, you go to Libby's. I'll walk with you." She remembered this until late afternoon.

I think I've discovered the reason why she repeats a question — "Libby is waiting for me, right?" — almost as soon as I've answered, "NO!"

She often forgets almost immediately!

"Sorry," she has a pained look that makes me feel guilty. "I just wanted to be sure."

Later in The Month

One morning, after breakfast, I went shopping. When I returned a half hour later, she was in tears:

"Thank God! Where's your mother? Who's your real mother?" She thinks I'm her granddaughter.

At 5:15 the following morning I hear Mom shuffling back and forth in her bedroom. What is she doing now? I hear a faint, "Libby?," then snoring.

At seven thirty she's in her bedroom, fondling her possessions. Junk jewelry and the real stuff are jumbled together on her bed. A gold chain, a gift from her sister in Italy, is so tangled that I had to break it apart.

"Do you want to get dressed?" I ask.

"I am dressed!"

She's wearing a pajama top, blouse, housecoat, party dress and black tights. Then I see what looks like a huge dark spider on the lower right corner of her pajama top. No, wait! It's her cameo broach, a pre-

Mom's symptoms fluctuated hourly. Most of the time she didn't recognize me, but occasionally in the mornings, she'd call me "Jo," apparently sensing that I'm her daughter. By late afternoon she'd forget again. Long after she started sneaking out to the yard to "make water," she occasionally found her way to the bathroom and recognized the purpose of a toilet seat.

cious antique, pinned precariously. She's smiling, wearing it proudly.

"Come, let's go down to breakfast," I gently lead her by the hand. She follows me like a child, carrying a wooden music box under her arm. Inside I find *my* missing bra, a stocking, a sock, and *her* blouse, all tightly squeezed in. At the foot of the stocking there is a small box holding her pink junk pin, and in the sock I feel the outlines of my pearl necklace — broken.

Eight-thirty, Next Morning

She's "fishing" for names, trying to find out who she is and her relationship to her family and neighbors. She doesn't want to let on that her memory is going fast.

"Where's the one who was here last night? . . . ." Her voice trails off. " What's her name?"

"Jo?" I suggest.

"Yes, I think it was Jo." Later, "Giuseppe, he's your brother?" (It's the name of her deceased brother in Italy.)

She answers her own question: "Yes, and who is the one with the girls, the one who is adopted?"

She tries to hold on to a memory before it fades away quickly: "You remember your father? His hair, it was?" She wants me to fill in the color.

"You're the one who was a little baby when Poppa would say, 'Come on! Hurry! Let's go to the movies.'?"

"Yes!"

As brain death spreads, the ability to recognize familiar persons and the use of everyday items is gradually lost even though the senses — sight, taste, hearing, touch — are intact. The medical term for this inability to process sensory information is ***agnosia.***

"Now I remember." Later, "I'm confused. Who died, my brother or my father?" She starts sobbing.

Next Day

"Do you want a hamburger for lunch?" I ask.

Mom doesn't answer. I repeat the question several times, louder. She moans instead of answering me.

"What's the matter with you?" I ask.

"What's a hamburger?" she asks faintly!

Mom has been unusually polite to me, pouring on the charm she reserves for visitors. I can't understand it. Is it because she finally realizes how much I'm sacrificing for her? No such luck! It's because she doesn't know who I am. Her eyes are vacant and questioning as she looks at me while I serve breakfast.

Memory of one's past fades gradually throughout the stages of dementia. Early in the mild stage, the sick person may complain of poor memory but usually this is not noticeable to others. Some gaps become apparent later in this stage although the person usually recalls at least one childhood teacher and/or one childhood friend. In the moderate stage gaps in remote memory become obvious.

Later

Without warning she asks "Who is your real mother?"

"You!" I answer.

"You're joking!"

"You're my mother! Why don't you believe me?"

"Since when?"

"Since you gave birth to me."

Her hands fly up to her temples; an anguished look crosses her face as she sobs,

"Why? Why? Why didn't they tell me this before?"

FLASHBACK 1928

The Rich American

One day Domenico D'Anna, who was then thirty-five years old and lived in the Little Italy section of Manhattan, wrote to his brothers in Petralia to find him a wife. He was fifteen when he first arrived in New York City, alone, with the equivalent of ten U.S. dollars in lira. Other than farming, he had no skills and he couldn't speak a word of English. Nor did he have relatives to greet him in what was then the largest, most cosmopolitan city in the world.

He had worked his way up from dirty manual jobs, at first cleaning railroad tracks and later janitoring in Broadway strip joints, to vaudeville stage lighting. When "talking pictures" arrived, he studied to become a motion picture projectionist. It took him twenty years to reach this pinnacle of success, for that is how his less fortunate paesani saw it. Most of them were still stuck in low-paying, unskilled or semiskilled jobs in construction or as street sweepers for the Department of Sanitation — the "Italian Army" as it was known then.

Since he couldn't be present in Petralia to look over its beauties, he selected his bride as one would select a girdle or brassiere from a Sears Roebuck catalog. He listed what he wanted:

- *Physical traits (big breasts were important)*
- *Good health*
- *Good family (no defects that might be passed on to his children, no taint of Mafia — an ugly legacy left by hundreds of years of invasions and exploitation in Sicily)*
- *And, yes, she must be intelligent and know how to read and write, for what good would an illiterate, stupid wife be in a city like New York?*

HONEY NUT CHEERIOS

Now, each week there is noticeable deterioration. Her memory lapses are becoming more frequent, and her learning ability is beyond hope. She forgets almost immediately what is said to her or whatever activity she's engaged in.

She eats two or three cereal breakfasts piggy-back because she forgets so fast. Her mind is like a flickering, dying light bulb. One moment she recalls Carl as her son; another moment he's her brother, Giuseppe, who lives in Italy.

"Are you my sister or my daughter?" she asks, haltingly, as she eats her favorite breakfast cereal, Honey Nut Cheerios. Several months ago, the memory of Poppa was still strong in her mind. It was Poppa this and Poppa that — how he took her to the best shops to buy her the finest clothes; how he loved her very much — on and on.

Now, at times, she seems almost to have forgotten the married phase of her life. She speaks more often of her "momma and poppa," how fine they looked dressed in their Sunday best, how respected they were by all the neighbors.

As the summer wears on, she speaks less of her parents and more of her "grandma" and "grandpa," even of her "great grandpa!" She doesn't recognize her father in a

Toward the end of the moderate stage of dementia, the sick person sometimes forgets major events in her past; e.g., schools attended, age at which she moved to present home, childhood friends or teachers. She also confuses the chronology of past events. In the severe stage, a few fragments of the past remain; e.g., country of birth or former occupation. By the final stage these, too, are forgotten, and the sick person lives only in the present.

Severe memory loss is not a normal part of growing older.

photograph and identifies her own photograph at age forty-five as that of her mother.

Is the brain degeneration gradually stripping away the layers of time, like a slow motion picture run backwards until the frames reach closer and closer to the beginning?

Two Days Later

"I am fifty years old?" Mom suddenly asks me.

"Do you know how old you are?" I ask.

"I was born in 1901!" she says emphatically. (She remembers the year of her birth but not her age.)

"You don't know!"

"In my heart, I'm young. "

"In your body?"

"I feel good, like a young person. Do you know how old I am?"

"Are you sixty?"

She laughs, "Ridickle!" (ridiculous)

"Seventy?"

She laughs louder.

"You're ninety!" I reply with finality.

"Never!" she shouts angrily.

"I was just joking. Are you forty-five?"

She pauses, not certain.

"How about fifteen?"

"Don't be ridickle!" (ridiculous)

"Twenty-five?"

"No, I'm not that young."

"Well, how old do you feel in your heart?"

She settles between forty-four and fifty years of age.

"I'M A PERSON! I EXIST,"

shouts a small sparrow of a woman at the Alzheimer's Day Care Center in Queens. She shouts insults into the air while pacing in circles in the back of the large room. The social aide put her there after she had punched another Alzheimer's victim. Like an increasing number of dementia victims, this one has been abused by her caregiver — her own daughter. The poor woman appears upset, as if sensing she's making a fool of herself. A social aide quickly puts her arms around her and strokes her face until she calms down.

A Tale of Two Cities

The old lady was found slumped in a wheelchair that had been left just outside the door of a hospital emergency clinic. There was a note pinned to her coat which read, "Please take care of her." As the nurse approached, a car sped away. The old lady had been dumped there by her stressed-out son and daughter-in-law who could no longer give her the twenty-four hour a day care she required.

In "A Tale of Two Cities," Charles Dickens described the nightmare of 18th-Century London, a city unprepared for the social upheavals created by the Industrial Revolution. Among the horrors he described was the abandonment of many babies and small children by destitute parents.

As the twentieth century draws to a close, we ourselves are caught up in powerful technological and social changes. Our traditions, social institutions and most cherished values are failing to keep up with a rapidly changing, electronic ally connected world. But we've gone one step ahead of 18th Century London. We have reached the stage of progress in which increasing numbers of abandoned and abused children have the company of abandoned and abused elderly people whose bodies have outlasted their minds.

I'LL LOVE YOU ALWAYS COME RAIN OR COME SHINE

Early Autumn 1991

At 6:10 a.m., on a crisp Autumn day, the trees in the back yard are ablaze with shades of orange, yellow and cranberry. Mom is on the back porch singing *God Bless America* as loud as she can. She's singing her heart out in the hope that neighbors will hear, admire her voice, and come and speak to her. Yesterday, I took her to a local restaurant for a brunch of waffles and sausages and she embarrassed me by suddenly bursting into song.

What a personality change! She used to be a dignified Sicilian woman who insisted on receiving "rispetto." Now she's an exhibitionist and demands attention from everyone within sight. Whenever someone comes to visit, she monopolizes their attention with incoherent tales of her grandpa and mamma, her "hitchy" skin and her daughter in Texas.

Later That Evening

Mom loudly accompanies a Frank Sinatra recording of *New York, New York, it's a wonderful town* with her rendition of *Santa Lucia*. She has been singing the same "toon" for almost three hours without pause. And when she isn't singing, she's talking nonstop.

I'm ready to crack up. Her grandchildren's maternal grandma, Nana, was in a more advanced stage of Alzheimer's, but she was easier to live with. She hardly ever spoke.

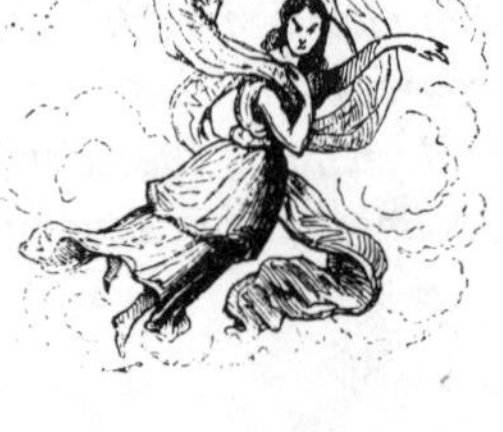

Culture and Personality

Anthropologists who have studied schizophrenia, which afflicts every society no matter how primitive or advanced, report striking cultural differences in the way the bizarre thoughts are manifested. This is not surprising, since many years ago Margaret Mead noted how cultural differences in child rearing help shape adult personality.

In Nana's traditional Austrian family, children were to be seen and not heard at the dinner table. But among the South Italian families I've studied and from my own experience, children are allowed to express themselves, and they do it often and loudly. If you don't believe me, do your own cross-cultural comparison. Take a bus ride in Naples or Palermo, and you'll feel like you're in the midst of a swarm of bees. Then take a bus ride in Vienna, Zurich or London, and notice the striking contrast. If you're the type who prefers silence while packed into a sardine can of passengers, you'll feel like you're in heaven.

All this leads to a thought: Is Alzheimer's manifested differently among different ethnic groups?

PROWLING AROUND AT 3:00 a.m.

Winter 1991

The temperature fell below freezing last night, but that didn't keep Mom from wandering throughout the house, sobbing and yelling at the top of her lungs, "Who's there? Anybody there?" In the morning I find her in her nightgown sleeping peacefully on the recliner chair without a blanket.

Night wandering is becoming more frequent. Now it happens almost every night. I used to jump out of bed at the slightest sound of her footsteps and coax her back to bed. Then I'd return to my room, hoping to fall back to sleep, but I seldom did. A part of my brain was constantly alert to her voice and footsteps in the dark.

> *Night prowling becomes a problem in some victims. Alzheimer's Disease can also affect the internal biological clock that keeps us on a regular schedule of sleeping, waking, and eating.*

"If you keep waking me up in the middle of the night, I'll have a heart attack and you'll have to go to a nursing home!"

I lost control again. It's one of the rare times I've made this threat. Afterwards I hate myself. I'm sure stress is the cause of the tightness in my chest that I never felt before Mom's condition got worse. Oh, what the heck! It's a good way to go, better than using a plastic bag, as Derek Humphries recommends in his book, *Final Exit*. (It gives instructions on how to commit suicide.) How long can I take this before my mind snaps and my heart breaks, I wonder.

"I don't want you to have a heart attack," Mom says in a small, frightened voice. Strange, she doesn't make any comment about the nursing home. Maybe she didn't hear. Blessed deafness!

Several days later, we walk past the new nursing home recently built on the next block. It's a warm winter day. Small groups of patients and nurses' aides are sunning themselves on the veranda. There are only two male patients, one white and the other black, and they sit close together, as far apart from the females as possible. The men stare silently into space, looking forlorn. Most of the women are chatting and seem to be enjoying themselves.

"Are you going to dump me?" Mom asks suddenly.

CONFUSING MESSAGES

This morning I put out Mom's clean underwear, *and carefully explained each item and why it should be changed every day.* There is no argument this time, thank God, and I leave her to dress herself. Later, I hear loud moaning, followed by a full-throated scream. I race upstairs again. She's trying to put on a stocking.

"What's the matter?" I ask.

"I feel alone in the world," she says with a carefully controlled facial expression.

"I won't baby her," I say to myself as I leave the room. I return several minutes later to see how she's doing. She's trying to attach one stocking to her garter belt with a safety pin. The other stocking is worn *over* her shoe. Her slip is tucked into her panties and the bra is tied like a belt over the outer garments.

My instructions were too complex for her to understand at this stage of her illness. There were too many words, too many concepts for her damaged brain to remember. I must speak in simpler sentences

THE SILENT KILLER

"Nice people want to commit murder, too," I hear myself saying. Don't get me wrong. I love my mother. She's been a wonderful mother, but maybe we've been too close. As a young, married immigrant in a strange city without relatives nearby, she had only me, her first born, as a companion during the day. And, until I was about ten years old, when I began to speak English fluently, she was my best friend.

But, now, after weeks of interrupted sleep, I fantasize about ways to kill Mom. Once I almost slapped her in the tub. Like a

> *Even once refined, polite patients may start cursing or saying nasty things. That's because the language area of the brain is damaged. Even though they want to say something nice, out comes dirty words because those are the only ones retained. The medical term for this is **aphasia.***

brainless puppet, her arms flail wildly about and her heavy body moves in directions contrary to my attempts to bathe her. And all the while she shouts in my ear. I feel like I'm losing control.

My brain seems to have compartments: one of love, one of compassion, but also compartments of resentment and fury. It listens to me whispering over and over, "Die! Why doesn't she die?" I just hope she dies peacefully, like her cousin Gracie. Gracie was enjoying a cup of coffee in her kitchen with a guest. As the guest dunked a donut into her cup, she felt Gracie's head on her shoulder. Gracie was dead.

Now I understand why some caregivers go over the edge. I find myself looking at the fresh blood stains (a result of frequent scratching) on her underwear with hope. She has been singing the same "toon" in a breathless, manic manner without pause since 6:15 this morning. How can such a loud voice come from such a small body? Mom crosses the line. She invades my physical, psychological, and aural space. While I'm sleeping, she enters my room and puts on the light. She barges into the bathroom while I'm naked. She sings and chatters incessantly and *loudly* into my ear while I'm reading or listening to the news on the radio. It drives me nuts.

The next morning, despite a good night's sleep, my ears still hurt and my nerves are frazzled. She's still singing that damned tune. Faster and faster the sound rushes from her throat, as if to pause means to die. Or, is it to confirm her presence on earth, to define her identity? Does she suspect it's vanishing? At this point I was not aware that I needed, urgently, psychological counseling.

"ROTTEN BITCH! DIRTY SWINE!"

Mid-Winter 1991

The skinny, gray-haired woman had been invited to join a singing circle at the elder care program held twice a week in the local Lutheran Church. But she repeatedly interrupted the singing with curses hurled into the air, at no one in particular. Instead of anger I saw deep pain in her eyes, as if she knew she was making a fool of herself. A social aide quickly hugged her and gently removed her to a corner in the back of the hall.

Some caregivers abuse their demented charges. Others abandon them, while a few see suicide as the only way out. Get help before you reach this stage of exhaustion.

I should be thankful for little things. Mom confirms her identity mostly through incessant singing and talking. Some dementia victims are angry and insulting, some even become assaultive.

SILENT STRESS

Three Weeks Later

It's now a daily struggle to get Mom to remove her soiled underwear and put on clean clothes. This morning she again announced that she was walking to Texas, wearing the clothes she had slept in — two "bloomz," a bloodstained undershirt and night gown, two pairs of stockings, an apron, a man's white shirt, and a flannel housecoat. Last night I was too tired and angry to prepare her for bed. She argues about everything.

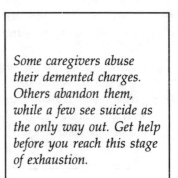

Our physical and mental health is most influenced by the quality of relationships with people we see on a regular basis, those who are closest to us. Relationships that are relatively free of anger, resentment, and hostility act as a shield against stress while negative interactions, if continued over several years, can lead to heart disease and a host of other ill effects.

"Take off your clothes and put this on," I told her, holding up a clean nightgown.

"I wear what I have on."

"To hell with you!" I mutter under my breath. I can't keep this up much longer. I try to trick her into changing her underwear, "Do you want to go shopping with me tomorrow morning?"

"Yes!"

"Then take off what you're wearing and put on clean underwear."

Again she starts to argue. It's too exhausting. I become angrier by the second.

"That bitch is killing me! She taking away the few good years I have left of my life. It's not fair."

Monkeys in a Cage

Long ago, in a psychology class, I saw a film that shows how symptoms of insanity can be induced in monkeys during a critical phase in their development. Newborns were each placed, alone, in a cage with a foam-and-fur padded wire "mother." "Mother" even had fake "nipples" that dispensed warm milk. Everything the infants needed — shelter, warmth, safety, milk — had been provided except love, companionship, and skin contact.

When they reached adolescence, they were placed in a large cage with monkeys who had grown up in normal circumstances. The normal creatures wrestled, groomed and chased one another around.

The "deprived" monkeys huddled in a corner, rocked back and forth, banged their heads against the walls, and scratched themselves constantly, like humans in a mental asylum.

WINTER ITCH

January 1992

Another thing that drives caregivers up the wall is watching the Alzheimer victim gradually destroy her body, and there's nothing they can do about it. Like many elderly persons, Mom has a chronic skin ailment — senile dermatitis. She constantly scratches until her skin is raw and bleeding. Within the last two years I took her to four dermatologists, and each one traces it to a different cause:

"Use petroleum jelly. With advancing age the skin loses its ability to retain moisture."

"Watch what she eats. She has a food allergy."

"Get a housekeeper. She's allergic to dust."

"Get out of town. She's allergic to New York City."

Finally her most recent physician, a gerontologist, admitted the cause is still unknown.

"It can drive you wild," said the sympathetic owner of the local liquor store. Her ninety-four year old mother also has Alzheimer's disease. "My mother constantly scratches her head. She pulls the scabs off and the blood runs down her face. I can't stop her."

She and I have become friends and confidants. There is nothing like sharing your suffering with someone who is experiencing a similar tragedy.

I suspect there is more to Mom's skin problem than bad air, withering oil glands, and/or allergies. I think it's also psychosomatic, a logical response to an existence without a future, without challenges or responsibilities and, like the deprived creatures in the psychology experiment, with little love and companionship.

CRACKUP

Early Spring 1992

A nervous breakdown can creep up on you when you least expect it. No matter how strong your ego is or how patient you are, it can happen. I was proud of myself for bearing up under months of interrupted sleep and the slow Chinese water torture of living with dementia twenty-four hours a day. The first time I nearly cracked up, in early February, I thought that ordering a copy of *Final Exit*, the book on how to commit suicide, was a logical way to escape from my unbearable situation. But I read that suicide attempts can misfire and leave the person alive and worse off than before. I hid the book behind the encyclopedia on my bookshelf.

"Why doesn't she die in her sleep?" I pray silently. I have a bad cold and a rotten headache. I'm neglecting my business and my income is declining so rapidly that bills go unpaid. "I could give up my profession and devote my time entirely to caring for Mom."

Severe exhaustion and personal setbacks can cause deep depression. One of the symptoms is "tunnel vision" whereby your entire being is so focused on your sad situation that positive ways of resolving or alleviating it are not even considered. All you see is a glass half empty. Getting away for a few hours of relaxation can change your focus.

For a while I consider the possibility of going on welfare and taking it easy for the first time in my life. The thought of becoming an economic burden on a society that wastes its human resources the way it wastes environmental resources gives me some comfort. But then I think, "Does it make sense for a person who is still productive to give up her livelihood in order to care for a walking zombie whose condition is irreversible?"

The round-the-clock care of dementia sufferers often causes their caregivers to lose friends, income and sanity. All I could see for myself was a future of even greater poverty, loneliness — and, possibly, dementia.

Mom's gerontologist phoned today. He had read my letter describing Mom's dementia symptoms. I also said the reason Mom seemed normal when he examined her months ago was that for the first ten minutes or so, it's hard to tell she's losing her mind. I also told him about my broken sleep and *Final Exit*. That did it! He prescribes a tranquilizer for Mom so she'll be quiet at night. His final words to me were, "I'm worried about you."

A STRANGER CALLS

Christmas Week 1992

My sister Libby died this week. We're waiting until after the holidays to tell Mom.

"I want to go home. This is not my home! My daughter, Libby, can take care of me. Will you take me there? You're a nice lady. I'll write to you. I'll send you money to pay for all you're doin' for me."

Every night now Mom now wanders throughout the house in the early morning hours shouting or crying that she is abandoned, lost, that she misses home. With her foghorn voice I can't get any sleep, nor can the neighbors. Two days later my brother Carl returns from the funeral in Texas. He's sleeping in a room next to Mom's. At four in the morning, loud banging on the wall jolts us from a deep sleep. Mom is stuck on the ladder leading up to the attic.

"I was just goin' downstairs. I'm gonna pack and walk home."

HER SON VISITS

Each time her son visits, Mom assumes he has come to "take her home." After he leaves, she paces about and makes little bundles of things to take with her. When we prevent her from leaving, she cries uncontrollably.

At 7:30 a.m., Carl is sitting at the breakfast table. He looks ashen. He didn't know how much Mom has deteriorated.

"Why must you try to do everything yourself? Why didn't you get someone to help?" He rants on, "Why this, why that...

"Can't he see I'm about to collapse? My mind is so fouled up that I misinterpret his feeble attempt to help me as nagging. It was too much. I hear myself screaming. I don't recall ever losing self-control so completely. I want to escape! I put on a winter coat over my nightgown and rush toward the door. It's bitter cold and there's snow on the sidewalk. At first, I had no idea where I was heading or what I would do once I got there. The subway seemed tempting.

"If you leave, I'll sell the house and you'll have no place to live. I'll have Muffin put to sleep . . .," Carl shouts after me.

He's losing control, too. Since he arrived from the Gulf coast, he has not had a good night's sleep either. He thinks his threats will stop me from

*The clinical term for such extremely agitated behavior is **catastrophic reaction.***

jumping in front of a subway train. He knows that I have a copy of *Final Exit*.

When Alzheimer victims are in the throes of a catastrophic reaction, it seems as though they are being deliberately stubborn and hysterical, when actually they cannot control their behavior. Their inability to estimate the seriousness of an event and how to react to it may be caused by damage to the brain's frontal lobe, the locus of abstract reasoning.

As I was about to step into the frigid morning air, I thought of Ernest Hemingway's father who left a horrible legacy to his children by committing suicide. In the years to follow, Hemingway, his sister and a brother also committed suicide.

What kind of role model would I be if I jump in front of a subway train? I recalled the promise I once made never to leave such a legacy to my beloved nieces and nephews. Although they call me a "weirdo" and "Dr. Schmuck," I know they love me and are proud of me. So, I went back inside, took a hot bath, put on clean clothes and came downstairs pretending to be calm and self-possessed.

"When a person is drowning, you don't sit on the bank of the river and give advice. You *DO* something to help save that person," I admonished my brother.

Carl was slumped in a kitchen chair. His eyes were filled with great sadness. He raised his head to look at me, and relief swept over his face.

"I haven't slept well myself the last few nights," he said, smiling weakly. He paused, "I said those things to scare you. I thought you were going down to the subway like the last time."

That's his way of apologizing.

FLASHBACK 1964

Where's Poppa?

My family got an early taste of dementia with my father. We didn't recognize the cause of his changes in mood and attitude at first. He had become uncharacteristically quiet and had been acting strangely since he retired. Usually when he's around there's a lot of happy noise: the old vaudeville songs, the rat-a-ta-tapping of soft shoe dances, the corny jokes, and the usual arguing over politics. But lately he's been silent at the dinner table. On this particular evening he was wearing his good Borsolino hat, and we were expecting another vaudeville routine. But his face was somber.

"Thank you for the delicious dinner," he said without smiling, "I have to go now."

Mom looked scared. "Where are you going, Dominick?"

"I'm going home."

"Where do you live, Pop?" I asked, thinking he was joking as usual.

"Petralia."

This happened more frequently as weeks went by. There was no way to prevent him from leaving, short of putting a leash on him. Physically he was still strong. Maybe a walk would clear his mind. The third time we called the Missing Person's Bureau, he had been gone two days. This time he disappeared for almost a week.

One evening we got a phone call, "Come down right away! Your father's in Bellevue Prison ward." He must have walked till he dropped, looking for Petralia. Pop had been arrested on false charges of trying to steal a parked car on St. Patrick's night.

One of the early signs of Alzheimer's disease is a change in mood and attitude.

"But he was lost! He was freezing and was looking for a place to lie down and sleep."

They ignored my pleas.

The infamous Bellevue Prison Ward was where they put psychotic criminals who were awaiting sentencing. Mom and I waited a long time in a dingy room that looked and smelled like a warren of bureaucracy.

"Come with me!" ordered a prison guard. He led us into a cavernous room divided by wall-to-wall prison bars. On one side stood guards in grey uniforms with guns bulging from their pockets, and on the other side a mass of huge men in prison stripes paced back and forth. They looked like killers.

"What's my father doing in here?" I demanded. "What did he do? He's a sick old man!" I yelled at a guard. My heart was about to burst from anger and disbelief.

The room was so tightly packed with prisoners that I had a hard time sighting Poppa. Finally I saw him — a small, frail old man, surrounded by monsters. He wore a striped prison garment, just like you see in the old Jimmy Cagney movies. His eyes were dead.

"I want to speak to someone in charge right away!" I was choking with anger.

After Mom and I arrived home, I rushed off letters describing Pop's false arrest to Mayor John Lindsay, Robert Kennedy, and the American Civil Liberties Union. A few days later, the Mayor's office called and a letter arrived from Kennedy's office offering help.

Multi-infarct dementia is caused by a series of small strokes in the brain. Unlike Alzheimer's disease, the symptoms appear rather suddenly. These days, it can be prevented or delayed with medications.

"Unless we do something, your father won't be the last senile old person to wander off and be arrested," said a lawyer from the American Civil Liberties Union. "The city wants to get them off the streets so the police can concentrate on catching troublemakers. We in the Civil Liberties

Union think this is outrageous. There should be support services for people suffering from dementia and for their families, not prison bars or back wards of mental hospitals."

Mom and I were eager to comply with any suggestion except the one he had in mind, "Are you willing to have television cameras come to your home while a reporter interviews you about what happened? This way the public can see what's going on." He also suggested that the ACLU issue a lawsuit against the city on our behalf.

Mom refused. The strain was showing on her face. Shortly after, she had a heart attack.

Poppa was quickly released to the custody of Creedmore Mental Hospital. Compared to other patients in the male geriatric ward, he was in much worse condition. He could not play poker or have a conversation with the others.

In those days, many people believed senile dementia was a natural aspect of aging. Old people whose memories were fading were dumped into mental hospitals where a special ward was reserved for them.

Early one morning, Creedmore Hospital called, "Your father had a massive stroke. He's dying!" I drove there alone. So withered, his body mass had shrunk to child-size. His eyes looked up at me briefly from the hospital bed, then turned quickly away; nor did he respond to my voice. I felt rejected. Then I realized he did not recognize me, that he had lost hope of ever seeing his loved ones again. I had an idea; I'd pretend to be Lucia, his beloved wife. Surely, he'd remember her. I kissed him on the cheek and whispered, "Dominick dear, look at me! I'm Lucia." His eyes turned quickly toward me, then jerked away again. His mind had played its last trick on him.

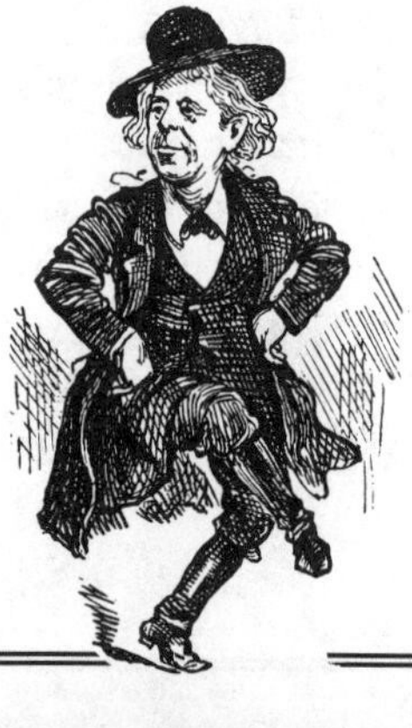

The Next Morning

A five-minute phone call from a stranger changes my perspective. Normally, I don't get phone orders on Fridays, especially during Christmas week.

"I'd like to order a copy of *Starting Over: You in The New Workplace,*" said a woman's voice.

Strange! Most of the book orders I get by phone are from libraries and organizations, rarely from individuals.

"How did you learn about this title?" I asked, trying to stifle the trembling in my voice.

The caller identified herself as a social worker specializing in gerontology.

"A gerontologist!" I shout. " A coincidence! My mother is suffering from senile dementia." Since my voice was still shaky from the most recent crisis, I thought I should explain. Surely, she would understand. And she did.

"Your mother has lived her life. Now it's time to live yours. Your main responsibility is to yourself," she said. "Your mother's needs are so overwhelming that you're in danger of losing your Self. Don't feel guilty. You are doing more than can be expected of anyone."

I could feel the tension draining away and the heaviness on my heart lifting.

"You need to get out more often and talk with people," she continued. "Join a support group for caregivers who are in the same boat you're in. Share your feelings with them. You'll receive comfort and advice that will get you through this terrible period. Put you mother in a nursing home and get on with your life."

It's odd how just five minutes of talking with a stranger whom you can't even see can change your life.

> *"Science has taught us to lengthen life. Now we must learn to make a longer life worth living."*
> *Helen Hayes*

"Did you call her?" I asked Carl.

"Of course not! Why?" I still believe he phoned the Alzheimer Association's hot line while I was taking a shower.

SWISS CHEESE MEMORIES

I simply cannot understand how her mind works. In some ways she seems almost normal. The memories are still there, but the logical boundaries of time, space, function, and kinship that neatly categorize them in the brain are dissolving. Each specific memory, instead of staying in its own logical compartment, is mixed haphazardly with other memories, like notes thrown into a shoe box.

Mom Meets Her Old Pal, Margaret Mead

Years ago, when Margaret Mead came to supervise my fieldwork in Petralia, she and Mom (who was visiting her relatives) were chatting on their way to breakfast one morning.

"I feel I have know you all my life."

"Oh, yes?" replied Mead, "through Josephine?"

"Not just because of my daughter, but also I have read your columns in *Redbook* magazine. Scuse me, I don't speak well English," Mom said apologetically.

"With your smile, Mrs. Danna, you could travel all over the world," replied Mead.

Throughout the years, whenever she needed a psychological lift, Mom would repeat that compliment to herself and often brag to others about the meeting, which occurred almost thirty years ago. But in her present state of dementia the encounter recurs in the oddest places and times:

- ▸ Walking with Mom through a shopping mall in El Paso, Texas where she is visiting her daughter, Libby.
- ▸ Dr. Mead and Mom go to a senior citizens' center on the Gulf Coast. (Mead was never there!)
- ▸ Waiting with Mom at the Dallas Airport. (Nor this!)

There Are Moments of Lucidity

Mom, who used to be proud of her cleanliness and sense of dignity, eventually became slovenly and shameless. She would not let me bathe her. She blew her nose on the curtains, undressed in the presence of visitors, and once wandered out in the street half-naked. Each dementia victim is different. Mom never made sexual advances, cursed, or insulted people. She maintained her ability to charm and flatter visitors until the final stage.

▸ Twice this week she dumped her feces into the sink. Yet she denies it even as I watch her.

"ANIMAL!" I shout in disgust. "Stop using the sink as a toilet!" I leave the room riddled with guilt and Mom in tears.

She's offended, "What you think I am?"

Later, I hear her mumbling, "How that could happen? I used to be so neat, so partickle (particular)." She utters a Sicilian word that means "work of the devil." The next morning, I wake up to find feces in the sink again! Mom is singing at breakfast. She had forgotten the trauma of last evening.

▸ Mom can still recall the main events of her granddaughter's wedding months ago — there was a large gathering, music, dancing, and she was the center of attention — but she does not remember where, when, or why.

▸ After we broke the news about my sister's death, Mom wept continuously for several days; then, as the awful memory faded away, she wept less frequently. Finally, the memory of her daughter, alive, re-surfaced and is still afloat. Every morning, about five-thirty, she shouts for Libby to "*come down* from upstairs!"

REMOTE MEMORIES FADE FAST

Late Winter 1992

There's a rapturous smile on her face as she murmurs, "This is the house I grew up in. My momma and poppa raised us children in this house."

Mom now rarely mentions her beloved husband. At times she denies she was ever married and had children. She often calls for her mother and grandparents, and she frequently lapses into Italian. Yet, at times she vaguely recalls an event that occurred that morning or the day before. It's as if a light bulb in her brain grows dimmer and dimmer.

Remote memory continues to fade relentlessly. In the final stage of Alzheimer's Disease, Mom will not be able to identify close family members nor will she be sure of who she is. She literally will lose her Self.

THE ADULT DAY CARE CENTER

The Following Week

"You *must* get away! Who'll take care of your mother if something happens to you?" The young director of the adult day care center looks concerned. It's barely five minutes since we began the interview to register Mom in her program and already she sees that I'm on the verge of another collapse.

"How can you tell?" I ask, trying to look calm.

"It shows in your voice, in the flight of your thoughts and your body language."

Right away, I liked her. When she speaks to the old people, she makes them laugh and feel good about being there. Her office is decorated with greeting cards from grateful caregivers. It's as bright and cheerful as she is.

Her tone becomes solemn, "Right now, you're being strong for your mother's sake."

The subconscious mind is a sneaky devil. It creeps up on you from behind and — Wham! — it knocks you out before you even know what's happening. I wasn't even aware that I'm about to crack up again. I notice that my hands are trembling and I'm sitting with my back turned away from Mom who has seated herself, as usual, too close to me. I hear my voice straining when I speak. Then I recall Mom's gerontologist saying, "I'm more concerned about you!"

The social worker wants to talk to me alone. She escorts Mom to the recreation room and returns to tell me wonderful news. There is help available for caregivers who, like me, are under an enormous strain — government agencies, private agencies, social workers, and volunteers who have survived the same torment.

The best news is about a respite center located in a private home nearby. It admits a limited number of dementia sufferers at a time to maintain a family atmosphere. The cost is

A respite center differs from an adult day care center in that its main purpose is to relieve caretakers of their burden for an entire day, a weekend, or several weeks so they can recharge their batteries. A day care program provides activities for dementia victims for a few hours a day, usually three days a week.

affordable. The bad news is that, as a new concept in dementia care, there are very few respite centers in the United States. There is only one in the entire borough of Queens.

SEEK HELP AND YOU'LL FIND IT

Let people see you're hurting, and they'll come running, as long as you don't lean too heavily on them. But if they see you as always being strong and self-reliant, they'll assume you don't need help even when you do, desperately.

For a while after my brother left, my nephews and nieces began phoning regularly. Despite their hectic schedules, they took turns visiting several times a week. The reason they had not done so before is that they believed strong and invincible Aunt Jo could never break down. One warm Sunday afternoon Susan took Mom and me to the Queens Botanical Gardens for a picnic. For the first time in many months I had a good time.

For more help, I phoned the New York City Department of Aging and the social service organizations I had visited with Mom earlier. With each call I got phone numbers of more people to contact for different kinds of help.

"If you don't want to put your mother in a nursing home, you can get someone to come in several times a week to help," said a man's voice at a local Alzheimer association. "It seems you only need a home aide now. She'll bathe and dress your mother, put on skin lotions, prepare her lunch, do light house cleaning and some shopping if you need it. You can have her as many hours a day and as many days a week as you like," he said.

"Suppose I get someone in the neighborhood. How much should I pay her?" I asked. I was ashamed to tell him our combined income can barely meet the cost of a licensed home aide.

"Seven dollars would be fair. Can you trust her?"

It was too good to be true. If I had someone in three days a week, four hours a day, Mom's social security check would cover it and pay for her medications as well.

A HINDU ANGEL OF MERCY

Late Winter 1993

Right away she realized Mom was senile and lost when she saw her wandering near the busy expressway. Thank God, Mom still vaguely remembered her address at the time, although she could not recognize her house. The last thing I expected to see when I opened the door was a tall, beautiful Indian woman, dressed in a silk saffron sari, with a red tikka mark on her forehead and a small diamond embedded on the side of her nose. She's about forty years old and, except for her cappuccino complexion, she could pass for an Italian.

Sukarma arrived in the United States less than three months ago, and already she has been accepted into a circle of American friends who meet mornings for Mass in the local Catholic Church. The fact that a Hindu attends Catholic Mass and that her best friend is a blond, blue-eyed woman from Puerto Rico hardly raises an eyebrow in New York, a city of rich cultural diversity.

Sukarma, who once was a high school teacher, is doing domestic work to help pay for her son's college education in the United States. "I do this out of love," she said one morning while vigorously mopping the living room floor. It must have been hard on her, an upper caste woman who grew up in a large house with live-in servants. Yet, she unfailingly arrived with a smile to help me with house chores. After Mom became incontinent, she even cleaned her soiled underwear cheerfully.

"How do you make peeezzAH!" she cheerfully asked one day. Like a mother who rediscovers through her child the joys of simply being alive, I began to appreciate again the city's ethnic diversity. Even simple things I had taken for granted were, to her, the most exotic of wonders — hot dogs, pizza, bagels, carrot cake, corn flakes, enchiladas, chili.

Within months of Sukarma's assistance, I became more relaxed and more affectionate toward Mom. Even my health habits improved. I had been neglecting myself, eating junk food and gaining weight, not caring how I looked, not even answering mail inquiries about my books. I didn't care. Being cooped up with Mom all day and night had become a living hell. Sukarma, a health nut, had a way of imparting little lessons on diet and exercise by using herself as an example:

A person with Alzheimer's disease can live twenty years or more from the onset of symptoms.

"I have discovered something wonderful, a low cholesterol egg!"

"Do you know that I drink eight glasses of water daily?"

"I walk at least two miles every day!"

While making these pronouncements, she would give me meaningful looks.

Out of Sight, Out of Mind

One day, Sukarma invited Mom and me to an Indian lunch in her apartment. As usual, Mom was charming most of the afternoon. For the first half hour or so, no one could have guessed she had Alzheimer's disease. Then, at one point,

Sukarma called me into the kitchen. When we returned to the living room a few moments later, Mom was hysterical, "Thank God, I thought you was gone!"

FIRE ANTS

Early Spring 1993

You can never look forward to recovery from Alzheimer's disease, no matter how compassionate and expert your care. You can never relax even when things are going well or when the arrangements you've made for assistance are working out better than expected. The only certainty is a gradual downhill slide.

Early one morning, after Mom and Sukarma had established a good relationship, and I had begun to relax in the belief that things were fine, she woke up twice in the middle of the night screaming, "Where's my brother?" (He lives in Italy.)

Mom always said she would live to be a hundred. Certainly, the genes for great old age run in her family. But now her brain, whose purpose is to protect the body from harm and sustain the juices of life, has become its mortal enemy. And it is winning the war.

Her body is on fire with many tiny wounds as though a thousand fire ants had burrowed into it. For days she has been scratching incessantly wherever she can reach. Each day she loses about one eighth cup of blood from the many tiny holes she tears into her skin.

It gets worse when she has no one to talk to or nothing to do, which is almost always because of her ephemeral attention span. When she has visitors, or if I give her simple chores to do such as peeling potatoes, she does not scratch, not once!

I can't do any more than I'm doing. I can't continually entertain her or take her for a walk to see her "daughter Jo" several times a day as she demands. I've tried getting her

Flashback: The Roaring Twenties On The Lower East Side

In Mom's hamlet, people speak the same language, pray to the same Deity, and share the same values. But, in New York City she has lived in several multi-ethnic, multi-racial neighborhoods. So, it seemed natural years later that she would cook a Kosher Thanksgiving dinner for a visiting Israeli friend of mine and, while in the early stage of dementia, invite Gypsy thieves in for lunch.

Her first view of the United States was from a fifth floor tenement window in "Little Italy," just two blocks away from Chinatown. She could see in the crowded street below a beehive of newly arrived immigrants from Southern, Central and Eastern Europe, all speaking different languages, some still wearing their Old World attire.

In those days the "supermarket" was a noisy immigrant parade of pushcarts, horse drawn wagons, and sidewalk peddlers. Pausing on every block, they would hawk their wares in heavy accents — fruits and vegetables, blocks of ice, yard goods, unpasteurized milk, live screeching fowl, household utensils, fresh fish, and other necessities of life. The air resonated with peddler songs in the various dialects of Italian, Yiddish, Polish and Greek. And, like an exclamation point to the ethnic diversity below, a huge electric sign, THE JEWISH DAILY FORWARD, blinked on and off throughout the night into her tiny apartment so that she had to sleep with the blankets drawn over her head.

Her next major migrations were to Northern European neighborhoods in Brooklyn where mostly everyone except Mom spoke English. By the time we moved to our present Queens neighborhood — where later immigrants from Sri Lanka, Trinidad, Guyana, India, Haiti and Puerto Rico refer to us as "The Americans" — Mom was already dreaming and speaking in English.

interested in simple pastimes like Leggo, Play-Doh and crayons, and knitting and making soap bubbles. Nothing works! Her attention span is almost nonexistent.

If she were living in Petralia, there would be many friendly neighbors and members of her large extended family to visit, and the time would pass happily. Here in New York City, she shares the same geographic space with her neighbors but not the same social and cultural space.

> *As the disease progresses, things the sick person can do become greatly limited. Mom eventually deteriorated to the point where she couldn't even follow the action on her favorite TV programs.*

She exists mainly in a community nearly one hundred years old which is buried deep in the recesses of her brain. Ancient memories residing there offer much solace. Still, she's a social being and likes to talk a lot. So she rubs away the top layers of her skin, sings continually, and talks incessantly into the atmosphere.

With her fingers moving mindlessly in a scratching mode even while she's at rest, she resembles a monkey scratching itself. Warnings that she'll get an infection do no good. Showing her the blood stained garments doesn't either. She denies it.

"Look at that blood! You did this with your scratching!"

"I don't know how that happen. I didn't do it," she says innocently.

She refuses to go to a doctor and screams when I threaten to call an ambulance if she does not stop mutilating herself. As each week passes, she deteriorates more noticeably.

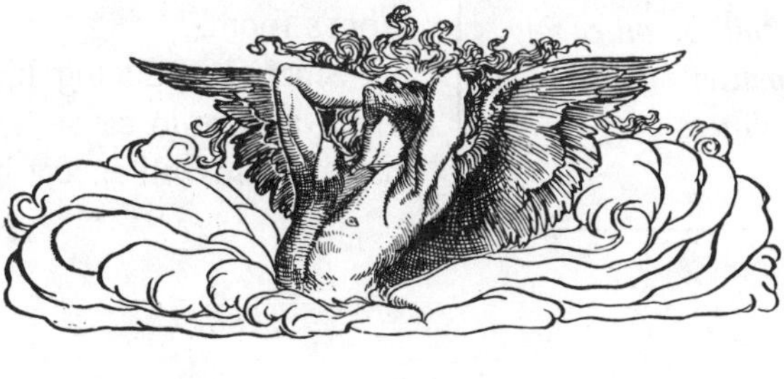

MOM'S "BROTHER" GIUSEPPE COMES TO LIVE WITH US

Spring 1993

"No! No! No! What if he comes downstairs with no pants on?"

Mom is furious because I told her a friend is coming to live with us for a few months. He has been over for lunch several times, but she doesn't remember him. She agreed the first time I asked, and he immediately started making arrangements to move in. Now, she has forgotten she consented.

"But Ma, he's only a friend. What can happen at my age?" I explain, wrongly assuming that logic can resolve this dilemma.

"Plenty can happen," she says, looking sternly at me.

She thinks I'm still a young woman and she is worried about my reputation. Maybe she even wants to preserve my "virginity." She's an old-fashioned Sicilian mother, after all, and can't understand that a man and a woman can share a house or apartment as friends. Mix the two sexes together and you get dynamite. It's nature's way.

Even in the later stages of dementia, the sick person needs support and understanding. Sven helps Mom retain her dignity and self-respect by listening without criticism or condescension. He encourages her to reminisce and express her feelings. This assures her that people will go on caring for her no matter how advanced her illness.

Sven is a college professor who emigrated from Sweden and is now a U.S. citizen. His marriage is on the rocks and he needs to get away for a while. I told him he can take my brother's room which is next to Mom's room.

Since introducing him as a friend is sure to cause hysterics, maybe Mom will accept him if

> *When the impaired person cannot remember things for more than a few minutes, she may still be able to make love, and want to make love, but will almost immediately forget when it is over.*
> *The 36-Hour Day, by Nancy Mace & Peter Rabins (Johns Hopkins University Press)*

she can place him within a family context. So I introduce this blond, blue-eyed Scandinavian who speaks with a Swedish accent to Mom,

"This is your brother, Giuseppe. He arrived this morning from Sicily. He has come to live with us."

Mom peers closely at his face. She looks confused.

"Yes, he is your real brother. It's been a long time since you've seen each other," I say hopefully.

She looks at him doubtfully, suspicion in her eyes.

"People change," Sven says quickly, saving the day.

That did it!

"My brother, Giuseppe!" Mom cries as she runs to embrace him with tears in her eyes.

Still, there is a lingering look of doubt on her face. For the next few days she watches Sven and me like a hawk as we each go to our separate bedrooms. Then, suddenly one day, when he isn't home, she cries out,

"That man is *not* my brother! Be careful! He's foolin' you. If he stays here, I leave. I go to my daughter, Jo!"

Several Weeks Later

Although Mom grew more suspicious, things turn out better. I try a new tactic. I introduce Sven each morning as "the famous university professor and author." This is easy to do since each day she forgets he's living with us. Mom is extremely honored to have this personage share her home.

Apparently she has decided we are friends, after all, and that her home is not be used as a house of prostitution. After several days of rearranging space and getting used to intruding into each other's routine, Mom, Sven and I are adapted to one another.

Mom seems happier now that there is someone else in the house to talk to and smile at her. She's also less of a pest because living with a "famous" man requires that she put on her best manners and courteous behavior. In fact, she even behaves more respectfully toward me!

Months Later

Mom is jealous of me. She wants me out of the house.

"Why did you come here? Why didn't you stay in your own house?"

She sees me as a rival for Sven's affections. She has even told a neighbor that Sven should consider her "better looking" and more "desirable" than I (am). She thinks he's falling in love with her because he fed her breakfast several times when I got up late and also because he's polite to her. No wonder she's been on her best behavior since he arrived.

Later Still

Sven has gone to Sweden for a few weeks, and Mom is unmanageable again. She's having another catastrophic reaction. There is more night wandering and wanting to "go home." Her fingers appropriate anything small enough to pick up. She puts odd things in her mouth as if touch and taste will help her remember what they are. Once she ate a spoonful of Vaseline, thinking it was food. She makes small knapsacks of clothing, toiletries and miscellaneous odd objects, including a roll of toilet paper, a floppy disk, and a bed sheet. Then she leaves them laying all over the house.

After Sven returns from his vacation, he keeps his distance.

MOM ARRANGES A MARRIAGE FOR ME

"You be all right if I go home?"

Mom speaks of marriage often now. In a subtle way, she's trying to get me interested in someone so I won't be alone after she "goes home." She apparently has given up on Sven who still lives with us.

"You was married?" she asks.

"Yes, once," I reply as I read the morning paper.

"Your mother, she was married?"

"Of course! Do you think I'm illegitimate?"

"No, I didn't mean it that way. I mean she got nice and married and she was happy?"

She repeats this question over the next several days until I'm ready to go nuts. At first, I take the meaning literally. Then, it dawns on me that Mom is hinting about my finding a husband so I won't be alone after she goes "home." Finally, one day when she asks again,

"Your mother, she had children and she was married?"

I shout, *"YES!"*

"WHAT! She married before you did? Shoulda' waited for her daughter to marry first!" (Often Mom thinks I'm her granddaughter.)

Several days later, without warning, she says, "When your heart tells you it's time to marry, it's the right time. Can happen all of a sudden, when you least expect. Don't worry. You find someone."

The dementia eventually infiltrates the language area of the brain. The medical term for this is ***aphasia****. Early signs are subtle. At first, Mom would pause in a conversation, unable to find the right word for familiar things. Eventually she couldn't carry out simple directions, like "Put the milk in the refrigerator."*

The Next Day

"She's a nice lady," referring to our Sri Lankan neighbor who, like her husband, is in her thirties. They're a happy couple with two children, "She raise nice children. How many, two girls?"

I answer "Yes," absentmindedly.

"WHAT! No sons?" she shouts.

Several Days Later

"The nice lady, she has a good lookin' son." (referring to the husband, who is young enough to be my son.) "You think he's good lookin'? He's single?" Later, "You talk to nice lady about her son? Does he talk to you?"

After several weeks of this I realize that Mom is preparing to arrange a marriage for me with Don.

"Hey, Nalini! You'd better keep an eye on your husband. My mother wants to arrange a marriage between me and him," I tell my neighbor. Shortly afterwards, I hear loud laughter coming from their porch. Nalini reappears and says, "Don says it's okay with him as long as the house is part of the deal."

FORGOTTEN WORDS

She used to be a nonstop talker. Now, the hallmark of her conversation is the incomplete thought, the forgotten word. Is this why she doesn't read anymore? Reading used to be her second great joy, after cooking.

She forgets words for everyday items like "garden" and "dog." Often, she doesn't finish her sentences and I have to prompt her. When she speaks to the neighbors, she lapses into Italian. She still sings, but not as often. Our neighbors used to love to hear her sing popular Italian songs. Now, when they ask her to sing, she can't remember the words.

DOES SHE KNOW?

Early Summer 1993

The great tragedy of Alzheimer's disease is that sometimes Mom seems to be aware that she's losing her Self. I'd find her weeping and saying softly, thinking I won't hear,

"I'm confused. Why can't I remember? God, please, make me remember!" — sob — "Better to be dead!"

Yet, at her great-granddaughter's christening recently, Mom was asked, "How does it feel to be ninety-one years old?" She replied, "Not too bad to be old, as long as I have my health and mind."

Victims of Alzheimer's Disease seem to know something is happening to their mind and their ability to do things. And, because they don't understand what's happening to them, their fear and anxiety increase.

Early one morning, Mom and I are sitting on the back porch enjoying the festival of colors in the garden. We swing silently for a few minutes. Suddenly, with tears in her eyes, she says,

"I'm sorry to give all this disturb'. If I wasn't here you wouldn't have to do all these things which I should do for myself. I never used to be this way. Please, I hope you don't think I'm cuckoo. I can't help. My mind knows I do things wrong but my body doesn't work right."

I put my arm around her and try to hide the tears in my eyes. She pats my hand that is resting on her shoulder:

"I love you. I love you with all my heart," she says.

"I love you, too. You've been a wonderful mother," I reply.

THE FLOWERPOT

- Mom can see a flowerpot, but she no longer knows its function, so she spits into it.
- She can see the toilet seat but "makes water" on the back porch when I don't catch her.
- She doesn't recognize the purpose of toilet paper and so she cleans herself with her fingers, then rinses the fecal matter down the sink or tub.
- She doesn't recognize her clothing as garments. She sees them as fabric to be cut and sewn. I hide all the scissors.
- She doesn't recognize herself, her husband, children or grandchildren in photographs. I had read that Alzheimer's victims enjoy looking at old family photographs. Since there is so little that Mom can do now, I eagerly try this activity. It's no use.
- Mom makes her own breakfast one morning. In her bowl she mixes water, instant coffee, two packets of Chinese mustard, and one tablespoon of petroleum jelly that I keep handy on the table to anoint her dry skin. I find her pushing spoonfuls of the concoction into her mouth with an expression of a child being forced to swallow cod liver oil.

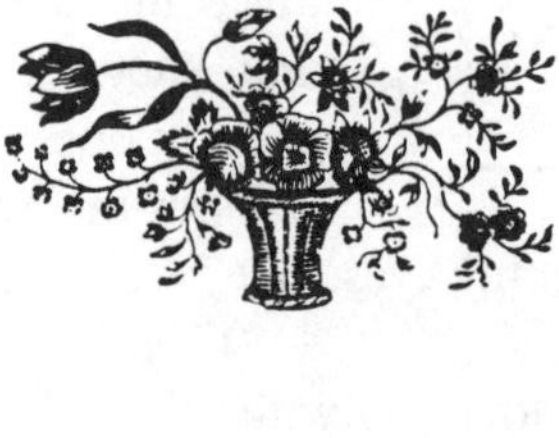

THE END BEGINS

Her suspiciousness is almost gone. She's more loving toward me. People tell me that I'm lucky; other dementia patients they've seen become abusive.

By late summer she's apathetic most of the time. She sits in the recliner for hours without moving.

Loss of locomotor ability is gradual. At first, Mom walked too slowly or too fast. Toward the end of the moderate stage, she took smaller, more tentative steps. Eventually, she won't be able to climb stairs without help and other motor abilities will start to deteriorate; e.g., sitting, smiling. Finally, she won't be able to hold up her head and may have to be fed with a pipette.

She's no longer able to distinguish between daytime and nighttime, winter or summer.

Occasionally, she rouses her memory about going to her house "where Jo lives." After midnight, she'll suddenly say, "Let's go to Jo's."

As I comb her hair in front of the large mirror, she asks, "Who is that?"

Mom wipes the crumbs left over from lunch onto a napkin and walks toward the back door. "I give these to the chickens."

She's becoming more unsteady on her feet. When I give her a sponge bath, she grabs a towel bar to keep from falling over.

BLUEBIRD OF HAPPINESS

The time will come when you'll ***know*** you cannot do it alone. At four o'clock one morning, again at the brink of nervous collapse,

I phoned the Alzheimer Association's hot line. Suddenly, I started to sob and said I wanted to die rather than go on like this. Imagine how the sleepy volunteer at the other end of the line must have felt.

The next morning a family counselor of the Alzheimer's division of New York City's Department of Aging called. She gave me the phone number of a psychiatrist who will admit Mom to a hospital for observation and a series of physical, psychological and neurological tests, including a CAT scan. She'll stay there from two to four weeks, enough time for me to regain my strength and sanity.

Then the Alzheimer Association put me in touch with several local social service agencies, one run by Catholic Charities, the other by a Jewish organization. I contacted these also.

Suddenly, all this help was converging on me. Mom and I were not alone, after all. People were genuinely concerned about our situation. Soon after, a nurse and two social workers from a local senior service agency came to the house. They advised me on how to file for Medicaid. They also began preparations to send me a home aide or admit Mom to a nursing home.

I then phoned the psychiatrist who had been recommended to me. Almost immediately, as if his office had been awaiting my call, arrangements were made to admit Mom to a private psychiatric hospital in Manhattan.

Mom enjoyed the "social life" in her ward. She was popular among the patients and staff, and when we visited her, she would introduce us to her "friends" no matter if they were fast asleep,

Lack of sleep, chronic fatigue and emotional stress can bring on one or more of the following symptoms of depression in caregivers: poor concentration, agitation or hyperactivity, decreased sex drive, decreased or increased appetite, easily tired, loss of interest in daily activities, feelings of hopelessness, thoughts of suicide.

drowsy from medication, or alert. Apparently, she didn't realize where she was.

The results of the tests to find out the cause of her condition, were not surprising.

"Your mother is in good physical condition but she has Alzheimer's disease. She's in a late-moderate stage and she may stay that way or progress slowly to the final stage," said the psychiatrist over the phone.

Several weeks later, the hospital's social worker called. "Your mother must be discharged before the end of next week. We're making arrangements to place her in a nursing home near where you live so you can visit her often."

"But I want her home with a home aide," I protested, still not realizing what this entailed for me.

"That's out of the question," the social worker said abruptly. She knew that in my present condition the home situation would be precarious.

I phoned the New York City Department of Aging to check on the quality of the nursing home recommended, and was reassured that Mom would get good care there. I also mentioned my wish to have her taken care of at home. Apparently everyone who had been in contact with the situation the past year knew about my fragile emotional state and the fact that, as a writer, I would not have the peace of mind and privacy I needed to continue my work.

The deciding factor was learning that home aides come and go and some of them may or may not be compatible with Mom or with me. "Who will help you take care of her while you look for and break in another home care worker?" I was asked.

Also, the advantage of having one-to-one home care for Mom would be outweighed by the many social activities in the nursing home and many people to interact with. In addition, there would be available a doctor and nurses, physical therapy and even a beauty parlor.

That did it! She was admitted to a nursing home where she shared a bright, clean room and private bathroom with another resident. The ratio of staff to residents was high and she was never out of their sight. The best part was that she was well liked by the staff and made friends easily among the more alert residents.

Mom adjusted surprisingly fast to the nursing home. "She's a doll," said several staff members, and I understood why she was appreciated. Some residents could only express themselves by cursing angrily into the air, and some complained constantly or slumped morosely in their wheelchairs. Mom sang songs in a loud, clear voice as a way of saying "thank you" whenever she was cleaned or served her food tray. In fact, you could hear her singing clear down the hall. This helped lighten the atmosphere but I suspect it gave everyone a headache. Since the staff thought Mom had been a professional singer (I did not discourage this belief), she was frequently asked to "perform" at social events. And when I brought her home for a day or weekend, she would stand proudly on the back porch and sing to an unseen audience. Her old neighbors would come out and applaud and shout "bravo!" which would get her started happily on another round of loud singing.

Music and singing enable Alzheimer victims whose language abilities are damaged to communicate and share feelings which they have difficulty expressing in words.

Just before Mom entered the nursing home, our relationship had changed to a more loving and compassionate one. At the beginning of her dementia, when I wasn't aware that she was sick, we were angry with each other most of the time and I didn't like her. Next came a stage of denial when I sensed something was wrong but didn't know how to deal with it. Finally, I read all I could about the sickness. This helped a lot. Most important was learning that Mom was not deliberately being mean and obstinate. Because of the brain damage, her ability to learn and understand what I said to her was severely limited. No matter how hard she tried, she couldn't control or prevent her behavior "problems."

One warm, Autumn afternoon, I was returning Mom to the nursing home after a visit to her house in Briarwood. I drove very slowly through the tree lined residential streets so Mom could enjoy the brilliance of November. The streets were exploding in bright reds, yellows, and copper. The sight was spectacular, and it took my breath away. But Mom seemed lost in a world of her own. "Look, Mom. Look at the trees," I said. She hardly seemed to notice. Then, as the car moved into the driveway of the nursing home, she perked up and sang, "Home sweet home."

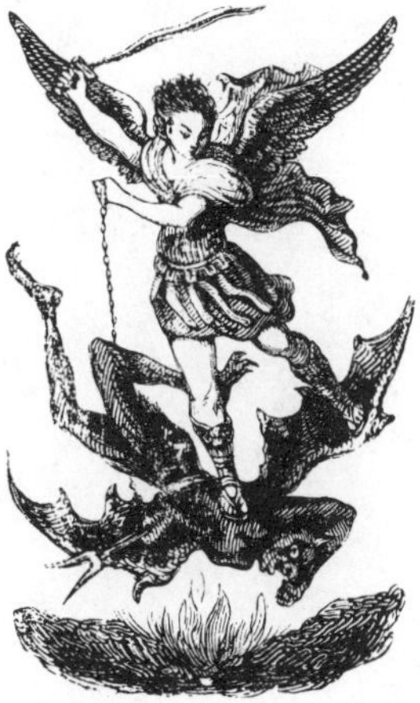

What does not destroy us makes us stronger.
Nietsche

Appendix A

CAREGIVER, TAKE GOOD CARE OF YOURSELF

No one is invincible. There is a real risk of caregiver burnout, maybe an eventual collapse if you devote so much time to the needs of a dementia victim that you neglect your own. The following symptoms of caregiver burnout are a loud warning to stop and think about your priorities.

- You often feel discouraged because no matter what you do, the symptoms of Alzheimer's disease keep getting worse, unlike other illnesses that improve with good care.
- You resent the time, money and energy your responsibilities are taking.
- You feel frustrated and angry when the sick person shows little gratitude and may even resist your efforts to help.
- You often lose patience and then hate yourself for lashing out at a very vulnerable sick person.
- You come down with colds, the flu, and headaches frequently.
- You have no time and energy for the things you enjoy.
- You cut yourself off from your friends.
- You show symptoms of severe depression.

YOUR PHYSICAL HEALTH

Good Nutrition Is Essential

Some caregivers skip meals and substitute junk foods because they're too tired or depressed or they have no time. They try to forget their problems by over- or under-eating.

Such practices are health risks that increase a person's susceptibility to high blood pressure, arteriosclerosis, cancer, and heart attacks. They also contribute to depression and anxiety, and they make a person look and feel older.

The body's capacity to store vital nutrients diminishes as we grow older. A well-balanced diet keeps us mentally alert. Studies link a deficiency of certain nutrients, such as the B complex vitamins and folic acid, to declining mental alertness as we get older. Low levels of vitamins C, B12, riboflavin, and protein are linked to lower scores on tests for abstract thinking and memory. Certain nutrients, such as the cholines found in dairy products, grains and legumes and the lecithin found in soybeans, improve memory in well persons.

What to do? Eat more vitamin-rich and high-fiber foods such as raw fruits and vegetables, bran, wheat and other cereals. Reduce your intake of foods that are high in saturated fats, salt and refined sugar. You'll not only look better and feel younger, you'll ward off hypertension, heart attack, stroke, arteriosclerosis and a host of other diet-related ills. The results will show in more effective caregiving.

Get Plenty of Exercise

You say you're too tired to ride a bike or jog through the mall? What you're feeling is probably nervous exhaustion. People who exercise regularly have more energy. They also sleep better and gain a more positive mood. Exercise gives them that "high'' which drug users get, but it doesn't ruin their lives and it lasts longer. Laboratory studies show that exercise releases certain brain biochemicals that ward off depression and anxiety, reduce stress, and relax tense muscles.

Fifteen minutes of light exercise a day, such as a brisk walk, keeps the brain cells and body young. It lowers the levels of blood pressure, weight, and cholesterol. Many bodily changes that occur as we get older are preventable, even reversible, with exercise. A 55-year old who exercises regularly and eats well-balanced meals can have a younger medical age than a 35-year old who lives carelessly.

Studies also show that regular exercise raises scores on various tests of intelligence and lowers the incidence of memory loss in well persons.

You're never too old to start a moderate exercise program. Ask your doctor what is suitable for your age and present state of health. If you have been inactive or suffer from a chronic ailment, starting with a vigorous exercise program may do more harm than good.

Don't Cancel Your Annual Medical Checkup

You are so rushed and so tired that you're probably thinking "Why bother?" But now, more than ever, you need a medical checkup to catch any stress-related health problem before its symptoms become noticeable.

KILLER STRESS

Do you swing between emotional extremes? Are you baffled by conflicting emotions? It's normal to feel grief and fear as you watch a loved one's mind and personality disintegrate gradually before your eyes and there is nothing you can do to stop it. In a way, it's like attending his/her funeral each moment. Grief is inevitable; we must live with it. But fear can be conquered with facts. Learn all you can about the disease, how it affects its victims, and how best to deal with it.

Guilt is another emotion that hounds some caregivers despite the fact that nothing they did or neglected to do in the past caused or contributed to the disease.

Resentment and even morbid thoughts are also normal considering the circumstances. Don't be surprised if at one moment you pray for a cure and the next moment you pray that your loved one disappears from the face of the earth. You're not crazy or evil. Such emotions and thoughts are inevitable. Get help before they go out of control.

Chronic Stress Harms Health

It takes a terrible toll on the minds and bodies of caregivers. Indirectly, it also reduces the quality of caregiving. Over time, it weakens the immune system and paves the way to sickness and severe depression. Many studies show that people who are chronically stressed have a significantly higher risk of developing heart disease, cancer, hypertension and other illnesses. Recent studies also link chronic stress to changes in the hippocampus (a part of the brain that coordinates memories), drug or alcohol abuse, domestic violence, even suicide.

Excessive stress also makes us less productive by diverting energy we need to give the best possible care.

There is also a normal impulse to vent our anger and frustration on the nearest scapegoat. Unfortunately, that scapegoat is often the sick person, as reports of increasing elder abuse show.

Instead of turning that energy against yourself or the sick person, put it to better use: Join a support group, find the help you need, learn more effective ways of dealing with behavior problems.

Alarm Signals of Excessive Stress

If you have more than one of the following symptoms, you are suffering from chronic stress:

- You feel irritable most of the time.

- You're always depressed.
- You have vague aches and pains for no physical reason.
- You have insomnia.
- You have dizzy spells.
- You're full of fears.
- You feel always tired.

Ways to Reduce Harmful Stress

Studies show that certain safe (and free) self-therapy techniques — cognitive therapy (see below) and relaxation exercises such as Yoga, meditation, and visualization — reduce depression and self-defeating ways of habitually responding to stressful situations. People who apply these self-help methods improve significantly, often as much as with psychotherapy. See Appendix E for a sample of audio and reading guides.

Set Priorities

A simple way to reduce stress and chronic fatigue is to limit the demands made on your life at this time. Do only those things that cannot be put off and those that are necessary to preserve your health and sanity and make the sick person comfortable. The others can wait.

Relaxation Exercises

Just 10 minutes of relaxation exercises a day reduces anxiety and depression, loosens tense muscles, and lowers heart rate and blood pressure. While doing the exercises, listen to tapes of calming background music or soothing sounds.

Visualization

This simply involves closing your eyes and imagining yourself in a peaceful, quiet setting — drifting on ocean waves, lying in a peaceful meadow, or any other place of tranquility. Imagine yourself seeing the sights, hearing the sounds, and smelling the fragrances.

Meditation

Meditation techniques, such as Yoga and transcendental meditation, involve the repetition of a soothing sound or relaxing physical movement to loosen tense muscles and calm frazzled nerves.

Biofeedback

This is a high-tech method of reducing stress and tension. Electronic sensors display on a screen how your heart rate, blood pressure, brain alpha waves, and muscle tension change as you practice relaxation techniques. Eventually, you will learn to control these physiological responses. Many hospitals have relaxation clinics in which biofeedback therapy and other forms of relaxation therapy are available.

Identify Self-defeating Habits of Thinking

Caring for a dementia victim can easily distort one's thinking and emotions. According to Dr. Blair Justice, author of *Who Gets Sick* (Jeremy Tarcher), often it's the person's habitual way of responding to stressful situations that harms health more than the situation itself. He helps his patients learn less harmful ways to cope with stress. One way is self-talk, to change the negative inner dialogue of anger, hostility, and pessimism that stimulates the brain to release stress hormones. There are ways to correct these negative habits with the self-help methods discussed below.

DON'T FALL INTO THE PIT OF DEPRESSION

Everybody gets depressed occasionally and for very good reasons: after surgery, a prolonged or severe illness, a job loss, the sickness or death of a loved one, a divorce. These periods of depression usually last a few weeks, many months when a loved one is gone. Even wishing death for oneself and/or the Alzheimer victim can be normal. Most caregivers snap out of it and get on with their lives and responsibilities.

But when simple routines become burdensome, like getting dressed in the morning or preparing a well-balanced meal, it's time to help oneself or seek professional help. Knowing how to help oneself and when it's time to seek help is what separates caregivers who get on with their responsibilities from those whose depression becomes incapacitating.

The link between mind and body is strong. Chronically depressed people have sluggish immune systems and are more likely to get sick. Moreover, they are much more careless of their own health. They smoke and drink more and exercise less than is required to maintain optimum health.

Chronic depression also decreases a person's ability to make decisions that will improve the quality of life. This is because decisions made during a state of depression are often based on distorted information and emotional reasoning.

Warning Signs of Severe Depression

The subconscious is a sneaky devil. When you're least aware, it can rear up and kick you in the behind, leaving you breathless. The common expression for this is *nervous collapse or breakdown*.

If you have at least four of the following symptoms, and they've lasted longer than several weeks, the first thing to do is get a medical checkup. Many physical problems and some medications mimic the following symptoms of depression.

- Do you have appetite disturbances?
- Unexplainable mood swings?
- Frequent crying spells?
- Do you feel hopeless about ever being happy again?
- Do you have bouts of guilt and feelings of failure?
- Do you find it difficult to make decisions and concentrate?
- Have you lost interest in things you used to enjoy?
- Is your sex drive a fond memory?
- Are you overindulging in alcohol or smoking too much?
- Do you have thoughts of suicide?

Are You a Depressive Person? Test Yourself.

- ***Do you measure yourself against a standard of caregiving that is impossible to achieve?*** Why blame yourself for a sickness that's beyond anyone's ability to control at this time? Just being aware of this can lighten your burden.

- ***Do you fail to give yourself credit even for assuming the responsibilities of caregiving?*** It's normal to feel frustrated because your efforts show few positive results, to rage against a higher power that has inflicted this terrible sickness on your loved one, to feel guilty about wishing for an early death.

▸ ***Do you have a habit of remembering your failures and ignoring your accomplishments?*** Inevitably, each event in which you fail to measure up to an unrealistic standard of caregiving reinforces your low self-esteem.

▸ ***Do you blame yourself when things go wrong, though there is insufficient or contrary evidence that you are responsible?*** You have fallen into the rut of negative thinking. You *can* learn more positive habits.

▸ ***Do you waste energy worrying whether you are doing things the right way?*** Try to view each problem that arises as a challenge, an opportunity to use your creativity and test your ability to adapt. If you succeed, fine. If you don't, try a better way or get help.

▸ ***Do you sometimes think this situation will never end? That the suffering will endure for the rest of your life?*** Join an Alzheimer's support group and you'll get help and advice from caregivers who have survived a loved one's dementia, who feel good about themselves for having coped successfully, who have resumed normal and happier lives. Think, "If they can do it, so can I."

▸ ***Do you sometimes think you are losing your mind?*** You're not crazy; you're going through a stage most caregivers have gone through. Indulging in self-pity immobilizes you at a time you need to take action, practice healthy habits, get help, and learn about the illness and the limits of what can be done within reason.

▸ ***Do you view yourself as a leaf in the wind, a passive entity with no control over your life?*** Don't assume it's too late or impossible to learn more positive attitudes and better ways of caregiving and dealing with behavior problems. Such a hopeless attitude might lead you give up easily or withdraw from opportunities for help.

If you answered "yes" to just one of the above questions, the activities described below will help.

HOW TO FIGHT DEPRESSION

Join a Support Group

You don't need to learn all of life's lessons the hard way. Listen to someone who's been there. — Ann Landers

During a recent farm crisis, farmers and members of their families were committing suicide at a rate far higher than the national average. A psychologist discovered that a farmer's despair was more likely to grow to intolerable proportions if he failed to discuss his predicament with others.

When we feel depressed, our view of life and of ourselves becomes narrow and distorted. We see the glass as half-empty instead of half-full. We fail to see other possibilities and options that are available.

We need the support of friends, family members, other caregivers of Alzheimer victims, and, if needed, a professional counselor or therapist to help us see things more objectively. They offer encouragement and emotional support as well as helpful tips on caregiving and how to maneuver through the health care and public benefit systems.

Caregivers who are in a state of depression also need to surround themselves with people who help them maintain a hopeful attitude and a positive self-image. Such people help a depressed person function better.

Alzheimer's Support Groups

Participating in an Alzheimer's support group can be as, if not more, helpful than expensive psychotherapy. Now, more than ever, you need to be with people who are in a similar situation. It's easier to unburden yourself of thoughts and feelings you would never reveal to relatives and friends.

Support group members also share tips on how to cope with stress and deal with caregiving problems such as how to prevent a dementia victim from driving a car. They share their knowledge about community resources, such as adult day care, elder law attorneys, nursing homes, and doctors who are up-to-date on Alzheimer's disease. Some also have a 24-hour crisis hot line. The social bonding that develops among members more than compensates for the isolation felt by many caregivers. There are fun outings, picnics, parties at members' homes, and other social activities.

There are support groups for people with special needs: spouses of younger Alzheimer patients, adult child caregivers, relatives of nursing home patients, younger children or grandchildren of an Alzheimer victim living in the home.

Meetings take place in members' homes, a hospital, church, library, nursing home or senior center. Many groups provide transportation for members who have difficulty coming to a meeting. Some have volunteer sitters who come to the home and some maintain a respite facility where the sick person can stay for a few hours.

You might resist the idea of joining a support group. This is typical. But, after you do finally join, you'll regret not having done so sooner. People at AA are friendly and sympathetic. They go out of their way to reach out to you. The tie that binds is mutual suffering. It helps to know others who have survived the nightmare of Alzheimer's, to discover that things do turn out better than expected.

(The people at the Alzheimer's Division of the New York City Department of Aging reached out to me. They don't wait for a caregiver to call back after the initial call. They know all about denial and resistance.)

Where to Find a Support Group

- Adult day care programs
- Alzheimer's Association, local chapter. Look in the telephone book under *Alzheimer's Association* or contact: Alzheimer's Association 70 East Lake Street, 6th Floor, Chicago, IL 60601.
- Children of Aging Parents, 2761 Trenton Road, Levittown, PA 19056. This nonprofit organization will send you a list of support groups in your area. Send $1 and a self-addressed, stamped envelope with your request.
- Medical centers that do diagnostic evaluations
- Nursing homes
- Senior centers
- Social service agencies
- Synagogues, churches, temples

Cognitive Therapy

To replace negative, self-defeating habits of thinking with positive, self-reinforcing ones, all you need is patience and the will to succeed. The following steps are simple to do.

Write down each negative feeling you have about yourself. Here are some which especially torment caregivers:

- I don't have what it takes to be a good caregiver.
- I'm too old to be doing this.

- I'll probably die of a heart attack or go crazy.
- I'm never going to live a normal, happy life again.
- Joining to a support group is a waste of my time. Nothing can make things better.
- I'll probably end my days with Alzheimer's and nobody to take care of me.

Analyze the logic of each negative statement. How true or false is it? Write down reasons for disproving each false one. Think of events from your personal experience and from what you've read and learned from others that disprove it. (This is a major benefit of joining a support group). Write these down, too. If you can't think of any, it's because you have a habit of negative thinking. Your pessimism shuts out other options. In other words, you're suffering from tunnel vision.

List your assets and positive qualities; e.g., skills, talents, courage, creativity, ability to adapt to changing circumstances, powers of endurance, willingness to take on responsibilities, family, friends.

Make several copies of the list and pin or paste them in places where you regularly look, like the bathroom mirror and refrigerator door. Read the list every time you get into a negative mood. Eventually your positive thoughts will become imprinted in your brain and the negative thoughts will go away.

Buy a book of encouraging sayings. Read several each morning as you eat breakfast and/or before going to bed. Here are some samples:

The gem cannot be polished without friction, nor (wo)man perfected without trials. — Confucius

Where there is no wind, row. — Portuguese Proverb

The only person who never makes a mistake is the one who never does anything. — Theodore Roosevelt

The most certain way to succeed is always to try just one more time. — Thomas Edison

Keep your eye on the doughnut and not upon the hole. — Anonymous

A clean house is a symptom of a blank mind. — Anonymous

As you dress or eat breakfast in the morning, as you walk to the supermarket or do other chores, repeat the sayings you find most inspiring. Mentally review the items on your list of achievements and personal assets. When no one is around, say them aloud so that they become more strongly imprinted in your mind.

Practice Other Healthy Mental Habits

▸ Each day, do at least one thing that you enjoy.

▸ Each night, read a few pages of something light and cheerful or watch a comedy on television.

▸ From now on compare yourself with what *you*, not someone else, have accomplished, and mentally review all the improvements you are making. Don't use an impossible external standard to judge yourself.

▸ Whenever you have an unpleasant thought, push it out of your mind by recalling the things that make you feel good, as Maria does in *The Sound of Music*. Psychological studies show that negative events or memories produce a chain reaction of negative memories, while happy memories foster more happy memories.

WHEN IT'S TIME FOR PROFESSIONAL HELP

We Americans tend to view our bodies as machines. We think first of tinkering with the machine, and we ignore the physical benefits of altering our psychological state. Sometimes it's not enough to get support from family and friends, to practice stress relieving and cognitive therapy techniques. If you have symptoms of severe, chronic depression, it's time for professional help.

However, a doctor or qualified therapist may decide that you also need an anti-depressant. There are safe and effective anti-depressant drugs. Such medications are helpful to persons suffering from clinical depression or when psychological methods do not work fast enough.

Many varieties of psychological help exist. Only short-term therapy is discussed here. This is because the stress-related anxiety and depression many caregivers suffer from are not usually the result of clinical depression or deep-seated emotional problems.

Short-term Therapy

Studies show it can be as effective as drug therapy in treating non-clinical depression and anxiety. Dramatic results usually occur after six to twelve sessions.

There are several varieties of short-term therapy, but they all aim to replace self-destructive habits of thinking and behaving with healthy, positive habits. There is no attempt to uncover deep-seated emotional conflicts. They work best on people whose problems result from chronic illness and personal crises in family, work, marriage or other interpersonal relationships.

Cognitive behavior therapy, for example, sees depression and lack of self-confidence as learned habits that can be unlearned. Dr. Aaron T. Beck is a psychiatrist whose success with this form of therapy has made it popular. He asks his patients to report or write down their negative thoughts, and then helps them discover the distortions in these thoughts. Exercises follow that instill positive habits of thinking. Often the depression clears up in a matter of weeks. The self-help tips discussed earlier in this chapter are based on this form of therapy.

Who Is Qualified to Administer Therapy?

Little or no difference has been found in the efficacy of therapy given by psychiatrists and other licensed professionals — psychologists, social workers, psychiatric nurses and pastoral counselors.

But be wary of persons who set up a psychotherapy practice without proper training and a license. Ask your prospective therapist where s/he studied. Then check the institution's accreditation. You can get help with this at the local library.

Cost of Professional Therapy

Some studies have found little relation between the cost of therapy and the quality of results. There are too many variables involved: the client's unique psychological makeup, the situation leading to a need for therapy, and the therapist's skills.

For **private individual therapy**, average fees per session vary according to the therapist's location and training. In large urban areas the cost is generally two to three times more than in towns and rural areas. Since the average length of therapy is twelve to fifteen hourly sessions, the following should give you an idea of what to expect.[1] Some therapists reduce their fees for people who cannot afford to pay more.

In 1988, private psychotherapists charged an average of $50 to over $150 for a single 45-to-50-minute session; psychologists, $70; social workers and mental health counselors, $55; pastoral counselors who have graduate degrees in psychology or psychotherapy, $35.

Group therapy is less expensive than private therapy. In 1994, the average cost nationwide was $40 per session.

Free or low cost professional therapy is offered by community mental health centers, university clinics, church centers, and family service agencies. If there is a fee, it is based on a sliding scale, depending on ability to pay. However, waiting lists may be long and the number of visits allowed may be limited.

At this time, some individual insurance policies have no mental health coverage. Others pay part of the fee. Some only reimburse visits to psychiatrists or psychologists. Generally, however, the coverage for outpatient therapy is not much.

Medicare pays half of its allowable charge, but only if the therapist meets state and federal requirements. The problem is that the allowable charge is considered too low by many private therapists and they do not sign on. Your local Part B Medicare carrier can give you a list of therapists in your area who are qualified as Medicare providers.

---

[1]More recent figures were unavailable at the time of publication due to the debate on national managed health care, which includes mental health care. The following figures, the most recent available, are given to give you a rough idea of the comparative cost of therapy by different providers.

Where to Go for Help

Relaxation Techniques and Cognitive-therapy:

▸ Community mental health centers offer classes and reading material.

▸ Many college adult education divisions offer courses and workshops. These are usually held in the evening and on weekends for people who work.

▸ Some medical centers have stress reduction programs which require a fee.

▸ There are many books that describe relaxation techniques and cognitive self-therapy. You can find these in bookstores and the library. Also available are videotapes that illustrate instructions on meditation, yoga, progressive muscle relaxation, and other methods of reducing tension and anxiety. See Appendix E: Where to Go for More Information

Low-cost or Free Professional Counseling May Be Available Through the Following:

▸ Community mental health centers, universities, hospitals, and health maintenance organizations can be found in clinics and non-profit private programs. Many of these centers treat depression, phobias and milder forms of chronic anxiety. In addition, **stress clinics** teach biofeedback and other relaxation techniques.

▸ Area Agencies on Aging

▸ Community social service and family agencies

▸ Many small towns now have therapists employed by the state.

To Find Licensed Private Therapists, Contact The Following:

- Psychology or psychiatry department of the local university, college, or medical school.

- The local Alzheimer Association chapter may be able to recommend private counselors who work with relatives of Alzheimer patients. It may also have a crisis intervention therapist to help caregivers deal with severe depression and guilt.

You can also contact one or more of the following organizations that have branches in many counties. Look in the telephone directory under their county or state names rather than *American* or *National*.

- American Association for Marriage and Family Therapy ☏ (800) 374-2638.

- American Association of Pastoral Counselors, 9508A Lee Highway, Fairfax, VA 22031.

- American Mental Health Counselors Association, 5999 Stevenson Avenue, Alexandria, VA 22304. Write for the names of certified clinical mental health counselors in your area.

- American Psychological Association, Public Affairs, 750 1st Street NE, Washington, D.C. 20002.

- National Association of Social Workers. Look them up in the phone book or send a self-addressed, stamped business-size envelope with your inquiry to 750 1st Street NE, Ste 700, Washington, D.C. 20002.

- National Mental Health Association ☏ (800) 969-6642. It has many local and state chapters. They may be listed under your county's mental health association.

- National Institute of Mental Health ☏ (800) 421-4211. For free information on the causes and treatment of depression and anxiety, write to: Public Inquiries Section, National Institute of Mental Health, Room 15C-05, 5600 Fishers Lane, Rockville, MD 20857.

If a Crisis Develops Before You Get Help

- Call someone in your Alzheimer's support group or the nearest chapter of the Alzheimer's Association. They usually have a 24-hour hot line manned by volunteers who have themselves survived this private hell and know what to say and do to relieve your despair.
- Call the local office of the Department of Aging.
- A local hospital may have a crisis intervention unit.

BE GOOD TO YOURSELF
YOU DESERVE IT

Stop Criticizing Yourself

Stop feeling guilty about the things you cannot do. Give yourself credit for all that you are doing. Pamper yourself. Be good to yourself for a change.

Take Frequent Breaks

Get away for several days. Even a few hours away from the stresses of caregiving will recharge your batteries. Find a respite center or a volunteer you trust to come in and care for your sick relative. Here are some suggestions:

▸ Treat yourself to dinner in a restaurant now and then. The change in atmosphere and having someone else serve *you* for a change does wonders for the spirit.

▸ Browse in the library or a bookstore. Window shop in the mall. Visit a museum. Walk by a lake.

▸ Have a picnic lunch in the park.

Make Time to Do Something Enjoyable At Home

▸ Steal a few moments each day to be alone and do nothing at all.

▸ Hide out in the attic or basement and read magazines.

▸ Make mail order catalogs your companions. (Pretending to shop was a great tranquilizer for me.) Browse through a catalog and mark the things you'd like to buy. Then, put it away for at least a week. By that time, you'll have a better perspective on whether you really need or can afford the item. Pretending is almost as good as doing it.

▸ When things get rough, order something you really don't need. An occasional treat is less expensive than a psychiatrist. It puts you in a better mood that carries over to your sick relative.

▸ Have long telephone talks with someone you like.

▸ Have fun with your computer. Join a computer SIG (Special Interest Group) and you'll be able to chat with instant electronic friends at your fingertips.

▸ Create something with your hands. Try knitting, gardening, sketching, painting a room.

▸ When you're too tired to cook and clean up afterwards, order in. Treat yourself and your loved one to a home-delivered Chinese meal or pizza. It's delicious and cheap and the portions last over several more meals. Why bother with cooking?

Make a Life! Keep in Touch

If you keep making excuses for withdrawing from all social activities, it's a sure sign of severe depression. Since caring for an Alzheimer's victim shuts you off from many social activities, force yourself to get out more. You say you have no time or energy to visit friends? At least stay in contact by phone. The telephone can be a wonderful stress-reliever. Use it often.

People who are socially active live longer on average than loners. They also have more opportunities to get valuable support and advice. Loneliness and isolation weaken the body's immune system. Studies show that having friends to share your problems with and give you emotional support helps you stay healthier and live longer. A recent study found that weekly support group sessions even helped women with advanced breast cancer. They lived longer, felt less pain, and were less depressed than women who received only standard treatment.

Now can you see the necessity of joining an Alzheimer's support group?

Get Help!

You're not the only one who can give good care. Professionals talk about the typical caregiver's resistance to "letting go." This fact came home to me when a woman whose husband was in the early stage of Alzheimer's disease called me for advice:

"I guess I'll have to sell my business so he won't be alone during the day," she said. She knew about various home care options, yet she demurred researching them. She even made excuses to avoid having his driver's license revoked after his two bad accidents. She hesitated when I suggested that she join an Alzheimer's support group.

She was in a state of denial. She gave plausible sounding excuses to avoid taking the steps needed to get help. She made no effort to contact the Alzheimer's Association or the Department of Aging for help in obtaining home care. She knew about support groups, but kept putting off joining. Yet, she planned to sell her weight reduction business because she was "too tired." At least she made a tentative first step by calling me, the friend of a friend. For some people, this is easier to do than to first contact an impersonal organization.

Caregivers need encouragement and time to feel secure about entrusting a loved one to the care of strangers who might not understand his/her needs. The best way I found to deal with this was to try it on a temporary basis and see how it goes. The results were far better than I expected.

Appendix B

WHAT YOU DON'T KNOW ABOUT ALZHEIMER'S DISEASE CAN HURT YOU

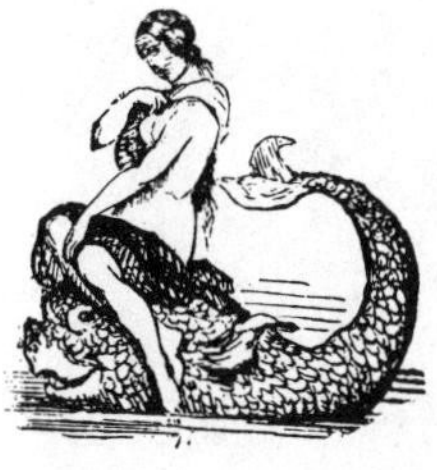

A WORD OF CAUTION!

The following is a distillation of several major assessment[2] instruments used by professionals to determine the course of Alzheimer's disease. As explained later on, a lay person **should not** make a diagnosis on the basis of one or more symptoms alone, because other health problems, some of them treatable, show similar symptoms.

A thorough and professional medical and psychological examination is necessary to determine whether a person has Alzheimer's disease.

Moreover, it's important to keep in mind that Alzheimer victims vary in their symptoms and behavior.

The following is a general guide only and is included in the expectation that knowledge of the disease as its effects the thoughts and behavior of the sick person will help caregivers avoid conflicts based on misunderstanding and improve their caregiving efforts.

---

[2]"Global Deterioration Scale," by Reisberg, Barry; Steven H. Ferris; Mony J. de Leon, and Thomas Crook. *Psychopharmacology Bulletin,* Vol. 24, No. 4, 1988.

"Brief Cognitive Rating Scale," by Reisberg, Barry and Steven H. Ferris. *Psychopharmacology Bulletin,* Vol. 24, No. 4, 1988.

"FAST" (Functional Assessment Staging) by Reisberg, Barry. *Psychopharmacology Bulletin,* Vol. 24, No. 4, 1988.

Don't deny the problem, as many caregivers do. Make an effort to learn what to expect throughout the different phases of the disease. It will lessen the shock of the unexpected and ease your anxiety about what may come next. It will put you in the sick person's shoes and make you more understanding and compassionate. Irritating behaviors will not bother you as much. You'll learn what the sick person is able to do and not do, and you'll find better ways of caregiving as the disease progresses.

This is an important lesson in giving good care, one which I didn't learn until mid-way in my mother's illness. In my ignorance, I focused on my own pained reactions to her strange behavior and I was not aware of the fear and pain she was going through. As a result, my responses were sometimes inappropriate when they should have been therapeutic.

ALZHEIMER'S DISEASE: WHAT IS IT?

Most of us will not suffer major memory loss in our old age, as people believed years ago. The term "senility" as a natural function of aging no longer has any medical value.

The true villain is a group of brain disorders that have a variety of forms and causes. Alzheimer's is the most prevalent. It is so prevalent that the term "Alzheimer's disease" is often used to refer to other forms of dementia in old age.

Alzheimer's itself is a slow-acting, degenerative disease of the brain. Ordinarily, it lasts from seven to ten years, but it has been known to last fifteen to twenty-five years. Most of its victims are over age 65, particularly the 85-plus group, but people in their forties and fifties have been struck down by it. Younger victims deteriorate more rapidly.

Incidence

Alzheimer's disease is a major public health crisis in the nation. In 1993 there were approximately four million diagnosed cases. By the year 2050, the number will rise to about 14 million. Not included in these figures are the many early-stage victims who were not diagnosed.

A recent study found the prevalence of Alzheimer's disease in the 65-74 age group to be three percent; in the 75-84 age group, nineteen percent; in people over the age of 85, forty seven percent.

Other Causes of Dementia and Alzheimer-like Symptoms

Is it Alzheimer's or is it something else? Alzheimer's disease has been difficult to diagnose with certainty, especially in its early stages. The mystery has been complicated by other conditions, some of them treatable, that show symptoms similar to Alzheimer's. A false diagnosis is not uncommon. In 1993, a simple skin test was developed which is highly accurate in distinguishing people with the fatal disease from those with treatable forms of dementia. It is awaiting approval by the Federal Drug Administration.

▸ ***Severe depression*** shows symptoms similar to those in the early stage of Alzheimer's disease — apathy, poor concentration, confusion, sleep disturbances, feelings of hopelessness, thoughts of suicide. It is now easily treatable with new medications that produce little or no side effects.

Many people in the early stage of Alzheimer's disease also suffer from severe depression. This double trouble intensifies the symptoms. Treating the depression helps reduce both the symptoms and the sick person's anguish.

▸ ***Multi-Infarct Dementia (MID)*** is caused by a series of small strokes in the brain that progressively destroy *various* areas of brain tissue, causing symptoms similar to Alzheimer's. A large stroke, on the other hand, damages a *specific* area of the brain, causing the loss of a *specific* function such as speech, form recognition, motor functions, and even death. A person who has had a large stroke may never develop multi-infarct dementia, although the risk is greater.

MID is easier to diagnose than Alzheimer's disease. The symptoms appear suddenly rather than gradually. There are peaks of severity followed by periods of stability and even slight improvement. Brain scanning techniques (CAT, MRI) can detect the destructive small strokes.

Early diagnosis and medical treatment is necessary to prevent further damage. The risk factors of MID — high blood pressure, overweight, diabetes, high cholesterol, and tobacco smoke — can be controlled.

▸ ***Malnutrition***

▸ ***Metabolic disorders*** such as hormone imbalances; e.g., hypothyroidism.

▸ ***Brain infections***

▸ ***Neurological diseases*** such as Parkinson's Disease

▸ ***Over-medication or reactions to drugs***

▸ ***Accident causing brain injury***

▸ ***Alcoholism***

Testing for Alzheimer's and Other Forms of Dementia

When dementia symptoms first become noticeable, to both victim and family members, a natural reaction is denial. This can make matters worse. Early testing might uncover another, treatable, cause and prevent the possibility of permanent brain damage. A thorough examination should include the following:

- *Physical Examination:* A detailed medical history and laboratory tests that include blood tests and metabolic screening for conditions like thyroid disorder and vitamin B-12 deficiency, chest X-ray, a spinal tap if infection is suspected, urinalysis, and electrocardiogram (EKG).

- *Neurological Tests:* These include tests of reflexes and sensorimotor functions; electroencephalogram (EEG); a computerized scan of the brain (CAT scan); Magnetic Resonance Imaging (MRI) to help distinguish between Alzheimer's disease, multi-infarct dementia and normal pressure hydrocephalus; a computer-enhanced X-ray technique (Single Positron Emission Computed Tomography (SPECT) which focuses on specific areas of the brain.

- *Psychiatric Evaluation:* It involves a clinical interview and an assessment of memory, perception and orientation, language skills, and emotional health. If the diagnosis is Alzheimer's disease, the assessment can identify symptoms that typically occur in the different stages of Alzheimer's disease.

Where to Go for Diagnosis and More Information

Alzheimer's Association

Alzheimer's Disease Education and Referral (ADEAR) Center, is a national clearinghouse on information about Alzheimer's for professionals, patients, their families, and national and state organizations. P.O. Box 8250, Silver Spring, MD 20907-8250 ☏ (301) 495- 3311. It is a service of the National Institute on Aging.

American Association for Geriatric Psychiatry, Box 376A, Greenbelt, MD 20768. Write for a list of members of the association who live near you.

Area Agency on Aging: Contact the local chapter or the National Association of Area Agencies on Aging, 1112 16th Street NW, Suite 100, Washington, DC 20036 ☏ 202-296-8130.

Private doctor: If you decide to see a private physician, don't assume s/he has training in geriatrics. Make sure. There are still a few general practitioners who believe "senility" is a natural result of aging or make a diagnosis of Alzheimer's disease without referring the patient for a full battery of tests.

For a list of private doctors who are up-to-date on Alzheimer's and other types of dementia, contact your local Alzheimer's Association.

Medical centers that have Alzheimer's or memory disorders research centers. They do research on the causes and treatments of Alzheimer's disease and related illness. They also provide complete diagnostic examination, as well as social services to patients and their families.

A medical center with a special unit for geriatric care and/or Alzheimer's disease has certain advantages. The diagnosis is made by a team of specialists in psychiatry, neurology and internal medicine using the most up-to-date equipment and diagnostic procedures. Some centers offer a second diagnostic evaluation and opinion for previously diagnosed Alzheimer's patients. Many centers have research programs on Alzheimer's disease and related dementias and offer free diagnosis for volunteers.

If the diagnosis is dementia, the medical center may offer a combination of the following services:

- Referral to other medical specialists if needed.
- Treatment of night wandering, agitation and other symptoms.
- Follow-up contact with patient and family, which may include home visits by case workers.
- Transportation.
- Day care or respite center.
- Psychotherapy or group therapy by professionals.
- Family and patient counseling by social workers and nurses.
- Family support groups.
- Assistance filing for financial aid.
- Referrals to home care, adult day care, and nursing homes.

To find the nearest medical center, contact the local offices of the Alzheimer's Association or Department of Aging. For a list of medical centers involved in research, write to The National Institute on Aging (NIA); P.O. Box 8250, Silver Spring, MD 20907-8250 ☏ (301) 495-3311, (800) 424-9046). It coordinates research on Alzheimer's and lists hospitals which are associated with medical schools as centers for the diagnosis, treatment and dissemination of information about dementia.

STAGES AND SYMPTOMS OF ALZHEIMER'S DISEASE

The following summary of the major stages and symptoms of Alzheimer's disease should be viewed as a *general guide only.* There is no lockstep sequence of symptoms that every victim inevitably goes through. Human behavior and brain pathology are too complex for that to happen. There are several important reasons for including this caveat:

Although most victims show the same *pattern* of deterioration, their *specific* symptoms may differ. One person may have delusions without hallucinations while another person in the same stage of the disease may show both. One person may exhibit restlessness by night wandering or sneaking out of the home and getting lost, while another person shows it by compulsively touching things or pacing back and forth.

The rate at which different patients deteriorate also varies. Even in the same patient, symptoms can vary widely within hours. (Some mornings Mom identified herself by her maiden name and insisted she had never married or given birth to children. By afternoon she was "Lucy Danna," a married woman with children.)

Another word of caution: ***Do not diagnose yourself or your loved*** one based on one or few symptoms. As we get older, forgetting things is the natural result of a life filled with many experiences. Our brains, like computers, can bog down occasionally from information overload.

Despite these caveats, it helps to know the general pattern of symptoms that affects most victims. It can reduce the anxiety of caregivers and help prepare us for unexpected eventualities.

Early Stage

Mild Cognitive Decline

The earliest difficulties are evident in two or more of the following areas of functioning:

▸ ***Recent Memory***

Major recent events are recalled with little difficulty, but the sick person may have occasional difficulty remembering *normal* routines of daily life; e.g., She forgets she just made a phone call and calls the person back. During a conversation, she repeats a question like, "What's today's date?" several times. Important appointments are not kept. Valued objects are lost or misplaced. Names of persons recently met are forgotten more often than usual. As a result, learning new things becomes more difficult.

▸ ***Remote Memory***

A few gaps in past memory are evident only with detailed questioning. At least one childhood teacher and/or one childhood friend can still be recalled.

▸ ***Concentration and Attentiveness***

The sick person loses the thread of what he's saying more often. When asked to count backwards by sevens, he forgets the beginning number or loses track before finishing. He returns from shopping with incorrect items and amount, has difficulty handling finances, and becomes confused when making change.

Complex games like bridge and complex routine tasks like planning and preparing dinner are now difficult. He may schedule a conference and ask half of the conferees to arrive on one day and the other half to arrive on the following day. Planning and carrying through an activity, like writing a business report, becomes difficult.

Co-workers often become aware of his poor performance before the family does. He may be forced to take early retirement.

▸ *Time and Place Orientation*

The sick person shows a poor sense of time; e.g., makes mistakes greater than two hours, or day of week greater than one day, or date greater than three days.

Although she has no difficulty traveling to familiar locations, she may get lost on the way to an unfamiliar location.

▸ *Language and Speech*

Difficulty remembering words and names are now apparent.

▸ *Motor Skills and Coordination*

Although the sick person has little or no difficulty doing simple tasks, *complex tasks*, including routine ones like taking a bath or getting dressed, must be broken down into simpler steps.

▸ *Mood and Personality Changes*

The first symptom may be a change in personality: A tidy person becomes slovenly and disorganized; a trusting person becomes suspicious and blames others for the consequences of his forgetfulness; a punctual person begins arriving at work hours late; a sensitive person becomes abusive; an outgoing person becomes introverted.

He shows mild to moderate anxiety symptoms.

Signs of deep depression appear: He is less spontaneous, loses interest in things he used to enjoy, has upredictable mood changes, avoids social activities where others might notice his deficits, loses initiative (doesn't start or plan activities on his own).

Moderate Stages

I. Moderate Cognitive Decline

▸ ***Recent Memory***

The sick person forgets major events of the previous weekend or week, such as persons or places visited; forgets the use of common items (tries to cut food with spoon); has a sketchy recall of current events and favorite TV shows; remembers little of what he has just read.

▸ ***Remote Memory***

Major gaps occur in recalling her past (like year and age of emigration to the United States, names of childhood friends and/or teachers), and she confuses the chronology of her life history.

▸ ***Concentration and Attentiveness***

Difficulties are now more severe: The sick person is confused by simple arithmetic, like adding 2 + 3, and when asked to make simple decisions like "Would you like apple pie or chocolate pudding for dessert?"

▸ ***Time and Place Orientation***

The sick person often forgets what month it is; often gets lost and/or forgets where he is.

▸ ***Language and Speech***

Vocabulary and speech difficulties increase noticeably throughout the moderate phase. The sick person talks less and her speech is slower, with many pauses. Her vocabulary is reduced. The greatest loss is of abstract words and phrases. As a result, her reasoning becomes more concrete. For example, she may interpret "Let's catch the bus" literally and say "Who is throwing it?" She forgets the names and functions of objects, and invents words as substitutes for those she cannot recall (like calling forks "spoons").

▸ ***Motor Skills and Coordination***

Routine tasks like walking, feeding self, dressing and bathing become more difficult. Familiar activities, like hobbies and carpentry, are difficult to complete and/or are done poorly. The sick person forgets how parts of common objects (like a coffee percolator) go together.

▸ ***Mood and Personality Changes***

As the sick person's failures continue to increase in number and severity, he avoids challenging situations, continues to blame others, and loses interest in things he used to enjoy, even television. He sits for long periods in one part of the room or paces about as if searching for familiar objects.

II. Moderately Severe Cognitive Decline

▸ ***Recent Memory***

The sick person now forgets her own address or telephone number, names of close family members, and names of schools she attended.

▸ ***Remote Memory***

Major past events of his life such as former occupation are forgotten.

▸ *Concentration and Attentiveness*

The sick person cannot recite the months backwards or count back from 20 by 2s or 40 by 4s.

▸ *Time and Place Orientation*

The sick person is unsure of the weather and/or time of day (doesn't realize it's past midnight and time to be in bed).

He gets lost when going to a familiar place; is unsure of his location (doesn't know what city he's in; mistakes nursing home for his own home).

▸ *Language and Speech*

Ability to understand written and/or spoken language continues to deteriorate, and instructions must be repeated often. The sick person has more difficulty finding words, finishing thoughts or following directions. Her conversation makes little sense.

▸ *Motor Skills and Coordination*

The sick person becomes unsteady. He walks slowly with small careful steps, bumps into things, falls easily, and needs help climbing stairs, getting up or out of a chair, and getting into bed. His handwriting is illegible. Driving a car becomes hazardous.

At this point, the sick person cannot survive without help. The caregiver must manage his financial affairs, do the shopping, prepare meals, show him where the bathroom is, help him take a bath, and do other basic tasks of daily life. Although he is still able to dress himself, he needs help in selecting appropriate clothing; if not, he may put on someone's clothing or a winter coat on a summer day.

▸ *Mood and Personality Changes*

The sick person is often agitated and restless: She paces, wanders, or compulsively touches things. Or she sits in one part of the room for hours without doing anything.

▸ *Delusions and Hallucinations May Occur*

Delusion: A false *idea or belief* which cannot be changed by reason or evidence to the contrary. (Mom's conviction that her lawyer, who is 50 years younger, is in love with her; that her village in Italy is only a short walk away; that she's in another place when she's still in her own home; that the violence on television is actually happening in the room.)

Hallucination: A false *perception* of objects or events. He sees, hears, smells, tastes or feels something that isn't there; e.g., sees the face of his deceased wife in a mirror, feels insects crawling on his hand, hears voices. Sometimes the hallucinations can cause him to harm himself or others.

Severe Cognitive Decline

▸ *Recent Memory*

The sick person forgets the most recent events. She doesn't know who the President is, but may recall his last name if given the first name. She forgets, or recalls only fragments, of her own address.

▸ *Remote Memory*

He remembers little of his own past, but still knows his name; can often distinguish familiar from unfamiliar faces, although he sometimes forgets the names of his spouse or children.

▸ *Concentration and Attentiveness*

The sick person forgets what she was asked to do before completing a task; e.g., when asked to count backwards from 10 by 1s, starts counting forward.

▸ *Time and Place Orientation*

He is unaware of his surroundings and gets lost easily, although occasionally he finds the way to a familiar location.

He cannot distinguish the seasons; e.g., puts on a winter coat in August.

His internal (biological) clock functions poorly; e.g., He cannot distinguish night from day, sleeps during the day and wanders at night.

He has no idea of the date.

▸ *Language and Speech*

The sick person fails to complete sentences, and repeats words or phrases continuously.

▸ *Motor Skills and Coordination*

She is unable to use eating utensils, and needs help in feeding herself.

She needs help getting dressed and undressed: cannot remember which article of clothing goes where, what goes on first (puts shoes on wrong feet or socks over shoes); has difficulty buttoning buttons and tying shoelaces.

She's afraid of, and resists, taking a bath. The caregiver must adjust the bath water, help her get into and out of the tub, and wash and dry her.

She needs help in toileting: forgets to flush the toilet and clean self adequately; has difficulty pulling up underclothing.

Urinary incontinence may develop in this stage. A medical examination might turn up an infection or other genitourinary tract problem. In the absence of such problem, it's due to a decline in cognitive abilities. Fecal incontinence may or may not develop. If it does, it typically follows urinary incontinence.

▸ *Personality and Emotional Changes*

Obsessive symptoms appear: continually touches things, washes his hands repeatedly.

Anxiety symptoms and agitation increase.

Terminal Stage

Now the sick person needs total care. Cognitive functions have gradually withered away until there is a loss of all memory, judgement, concentration, speech, basic motor skills and, finally, consciousness.

▸ *Loss of Verbal Abilities*

The sick person no longer understands what others are saying. She may be able to repeat words or simple phrases but does not understand their meaning. Eventually, she loses the ability to speak entirely or her vocabulary is limited to one or two words that are repeated continuously and used to express every need. Finally, there is no speech at all, only grunts and screams.

▸ *Loss of Basic Psychomotor Skills*

Ability to smile, walk, sit, hold head up, and even swallow food is gradually lost. Finally, the sick person loses consciousness.

Appendix C

HELP FOR CAREGIVERS

You have a choice among different kinds of services and where they are provided — in your own home, a community organization, or a long-term care facility. The following overview will help you decide which services are best for you at this time and which ones to plan for as your loved one's sickness progresses.

VOLUNTEER HELP

At first, many caregivers think they can handle everything by themselves — taking care of the sick person and getting information on home care, adult day care, nursing homes, legal resources, eligibility for Medicaid and other public benefits. (I did, before I got wiser. Neither I nor my family expected it to be such a demanding, full time job.

(Even after my need for help became critical, I made the mistake of waiting for it to be offered to me. If I had shared what I knew about Alzheimer's disease with my family, neighbors, and friends, they would have understood the reason for Mom's strange behavior and how frustrating and exhausting caregiving can be. A neighbor would not have called the police at 4:00 a.m. one morning, on the mistaken assumption that Mom was screaming because I was abusing her.

(I didn't realize people were waiting for me to make the first move. I should have called a family meeting so we could plan together how to share tasks I could no longer do on my own.

Social psychology studies show that people are more likely to carry out their offer to help when it is made before an audience. It's also easier that way to set up a schedule of how much time each volunteer can give and when.)

Some Ways Volunteers Can Help

- Make phone calls and/or visits to learn about community resources and eligibility requirements.
- Take turns a few hours a week or month staying with the sick relative so you can get out and recharge your batteries.
- Drive the sick person to appointments.
- Shop for groceries and do other errands.
- Handle forms and financial matters.
- Consult with medical and legal experts.
- Those who have no time to give may offer to share the cost of hiring a home care worker.

Sources of Volunteer Help

In addition to family, friends and neighbors, there are community sources of volunteer help; e.g., senior centers; churches and synagogues; local ethnic, fraternal and religious associations; local Alzheimer Association chapters; local agencies on aging; American Association of Retired persons (more below).

HOME CARE

Home care enables you to keep your loved one at home longer. It also gives you more time to rest and carry on with your own life, even keep a job. The services range from help with household tasks and meal preparation to specialized health services. The hours of service can range from several a week to round-the-clock care. In 1993, families spent an average of $18,000 on home care for an Alzheimer's victim.[3]

Meals on Wheels

This service provides volunteers who deliver one hot meal a day to homebound elderly persons who live alone. The brief visit is also a much needed social occasion. If a sick relative lives far away, it's reassuring to know someone will visit daily to make sure s/he is all right.

Information on how to apply for this service can be obtained from local chapters of the Alzheimer's Association, AARP (American Association of Retired Persons), Department of Aging, and Area Agencies on Aging. The service costs very little and is free for persons who met the income eligibility test.

Senior Companions

This is a nationwide program in which volunteers, typically senior citizens, take the sick person out for walks and encourage her to do exercises, games and other activities. The local chapters of the American Association of Retired Persons and the Alzheimer Association can refer you to a Senior Companion Program.

---

[3]This and the following figures on various types of home care are the most recent I could find during this period of hot political debate on managed health care. You are advised to make a comparison of current health care costs in your community from figures provided by the local Alzheimer's Association, Department of Aging, and various private homecare agencies.

Home Aides

They are paid, part-time workers who do light housekeeping, shopping and meal preparation; escort frail persons to medical appointments; and other supportive services. In 1993 the average cost was $40 to $60, plus lunch, for a three-to-four hour visit depending on the region. A freelance home aide typically charged $6 per hour.

Home Health Aides

They have more advanced duties like changing dressings, supervising baths and physical therapy, and reminding the sick person to take medication. In 1993 the annual average cost was $14 to $17 per hour depending on the region.[4] Medicaid helps in some states.

Visiting Registered Nurses and Licensed Practical Nurses

They oversee the sick person's pulse and blood pressure, administer medication and therapy, and give other types of professional health care. If your sick relative lives alone, you can hire a nurse to visit regularly. The nurse will monitor his health, carry out doctor's orders, prepare medications, and supervise the care given by a home aide. The annual average cost in 1993 was $60 to $80 for a three-to-four hour visit, depending on the region.

---

[4]In 1993, New York City, a home health-care worker who also provided medical attention cost $31,000 annually.

Long-term Home Care

This service can be expensive. In 1993 for example, a four-hour -day, five-day-week home care aide cost $8,000 to $14,000 a year on average. In high-cost areas like New York City, a family could spend $30,000 a year or more. One financially strapped caregiver who had a full-time job and needed round-the-clock care for her mother reduced expenses by furnishing a small apartment in the basement and hiring a live-in home care worker, with full room and board provided.

You can probably find a home care worker who will provide several kinds of care described above: a home aide to help your relative bathe and dress, as well as prepare meals, do light shopping, provide exercise and other activities, and escort him to medical appointments.

Where to Find Home Care

▸ The Alzheimer's Unit of the local Department for the Aging offers counseling and information to help you get home care as well as information on Medicaid eligibility for home care and how to apply.

▸ In some areas, the Alzheimer's Association works with Medicaid funded and private home care agencies to train aides to work with dementia victims. Some chapters also help families navigate through the bureaucratic maze of applying for public services.

▸ Geriatric centers associated with universities or hospitals.

▸ Local senior service organizations: The New York Foundation for Senior Citizens in New York City, for example, has a program that offers personal care, meal preparation, shopping, escort services, and light housekeeping and laundry. Service is provided for a maximum time of three months; the minimum is twice a week, four hours per visit. Fees in 1993 were $6.00 per hour on weekdays and $6.50 on weekends.

▸ Private agencies: Since, ideally, they have already checked the recommendations and experience of persons whom they hire, they'll save you the time and effort in doing your own background check. They'll also save you time in supervision and paperwork. There is a fee for this service. Look in the Yellow Pages under *Senior . . .*, *Geriatric . . .*, *Home Care . . .* , and compare fees.

If your loved one has an additional health problem, you can get long-term home health care from a professional agency. Many of these are run by registered nurses.

▸ Nursing homes: Look for those that have long-term home health care programs. These typically provide a combination of the following services: dieticians for nutritional counseling; delivery of hot meals, medical supplies and equipment; home health aides; licensed nurses to visit your relative regularly; physical and respiratory therapists who come to the home; social workers to help you find other caregiving options and apply for public benefits; telephone hot lines that offer advice on health and service related emergencies; transportation to medical appointments.

▸ There are also many freelance home care aides. You can find their notices posted on neighborhood bulletin boards and in local newspapers. The local Alzheimer's support group and the Department of Aging are good sources of reliable freelance help. Senior centers also can provide names of freelancers who have been recommended by participants.

Before hiring someone you don't know, ask about her training and experience. Make a thorough background check and contact all references. Ask for referrals from other people who have used home care.

Consult with the Alzheimer's Association and the Department of Aging on how to supervise and evaluate the worker's performance. Another source of information is *Beat the Nursing Home Trap* by Joseph Matthews (Nolo Press, Berkeley. 1994)

Also, it's wise to prepare in advance for the days when your aide is absent, either because of illness or some other reason.

▸ *Older Americans Act (OAA) programs* are available to all persons 60 years of age or older. Some are for low income persons only. The services include Visiting Nurses, Meals on Wheels, and home repair. These are available through the local Area Agency on Aging, senior centers, social service agencies, and religious organizations.

ADULT DAY CARE

Adult day care provides family caregivers with much needed relief for several hours a day, several days a week. Unlike typical senior centers, the participants receive more supervision and activities are adapted to their special needs.

Hours of attendance range from three to twelve hours a day and from two to seven days a week, depending on the facility. Most centers provide lunch.

Services range from simple recreation and socialization activities to rehabilitation and health care provided by professionals. The activities include any or all of the following: arts and crafts, group singing, discussion groups, exercises, gardening, picnics and outings. Probably the most valuable service of all is to offer the frail participants an opportunity to socialize.

Admission requirements vary. At present, many day care centers do not admit persons with *advanced* Alzheimer's disease. However, an increasing number are developing special programs for victims who are in the *early* stages of the disease. These programs provide more personal care from specially trained aides and have activities designed to stimulate social and cognitive abilities.

Adult Day Care Centers Associated with Nursing Homes

These generally have two separate programs, one for persons with mild to moderate dementia and the other for persons with severe dementia. The hours generally run from five to six hours a day, seven days a week.

Services

In addition to the usual social and recreational activities and a hot meal, they include any or all of the following:

▸ Rehabilitation and health services: physical therapy, audiology, nursing, dental, podiatry, assistance with toileting and feeding, blood pressure checks, administering medications, and changing dressings.

▸ A dietician and/or nurse to advise caregivers on good nutrition and how to care for the sick person at home.

▸ A social worker who provides referrals to other community resources and information on how to apply for financial aid, where to get expert counsel on the legal transfer of assets and property, and how to apply for nursing home care.

▸ Support groups for families.

▸ Transportation to and from the center, in some cases by buses with wheelchair lifts.

▸ Special diets.

▸ An additional advantage is that it makes eventual long-term care placement less traumatic for the sick person and the family.

Some day care centers accept Medicaid. Some merely ask for a voluntary contribution. Many of the more expensive ones have a sliding scale of fees based on ability to pay.

Admission Requirements

Until recently, most adult day care programs did not have special provisions for Alzheimer victims and many still refuse to admit them, especially persons in an advanced stage of the disease. The good news is that, as a result of a growing national need, there will be more adult day care centers with special programs for Alzheimer victims.

Some, while not intended for dementia sufferers, will admit persons in the early stages of Alzheimer's. Generally, they require that the person have manageable incontinence and wandering behavior, and can feed herself and function within a group. Some centers will admit persons who are beyond the moderate stage as long a home caregiver is present.

Where to Find Adult Day Care Centers

▸ Churches, synagogues, temples

▸ Community sponsored programs (contact your local Alzheimer's Association and public library).

▸ Geriatric centers affiliated with hospitals and medical schools.

▸ Medical centers with a geriatric program.

▸ Nursing homes that have short-stay respite programs.

▸ Religion affiliated agencies.

▸ Senior citizen organizations.

In addition to the sources listed above, contact the following for a list of centers located near you:

▸ Adult Day Services Association in your state.

▸ The National Institute on Adult Day Care, 600 Maryland Avenue, SW, West Wing 100, Washington, DC 20024 ☏ (202) 479-1200.

▸ The National Council on Aging has a toll-free referral service ☏ (800) 424-9046, [residents of Maryland, Virginia and Washington, D.C. ☏ (202) 479-1200].

RESPITE CARE

Respite care can be provided in the patient's own home or in respite care centers located in churches, community centers, private homes, and nursing homes.

Respite Centers

Unlike adult day care centers which operate a few hours a day, several days a week, respite centers offer longer-term temporary care. You can leave your sick relative there for a whole day, several overnight stays, even weeks at a time.

Respite centers are a relatively new service. At present few exist in many communities, and most of these were established only within the last few years.

Services

In addition to personal care, some respite centers provide social and recreational activities for their impaired guests. Some also provide door-to-door transportation.

At present, the quality and extent of services vary widely. Some centers just babysit. Others, especially those run by hospital geriatric units and nursing homes, offer a full range of services. The following notes come from a brochure for a respite care center offered by a nursing home affiliated with a religious organization:

Individualized programs are tailored to each "guest's" special needs, tastes, abilities, and ethnic and religious affiliation. Volunteers are recruited who understand their language and culture. In addition to providing for each guest's social, recreational, medical, nursing and dietary needs, a personal physician is assigned and there is 24-hour nursing care. The guests can also participate in the regular activities of the nursing home: arts and crafts, games, movies, musical events, parties, trips, physical fitness activities. Family caregivers are offered legal and personal counseling services, support groups, educational lectures on how to manage Alzheimer patients at home, and a lending library on dementia disorders.

The physical setting can also vary widely. "Guests" in this center stay in attractively furnished double rooms with private bathrooms, with full housekeeping services provided. Single rooms are available for guests with special needs. By way of contrast, a center I visited was located near an industrial area that was difficult to get to. A tiny back porch faced a brick wall and the "yard" was a small concrete block. Rooms were dark even on a sunny day. As if to compensate for this, the cost was very reasonable.

Admission Requirements

At present, there is a severe shortage of respite centers. Reservations should be made at least four weeks up to a year in advance.

Ideally, the admissions procedure should include a review of the sick person's social and medical history: hobbies and interests, work history, current level of functioning, a recent health examination. At least one family member should be readily available by phone and direct contact.

Cost

It can range from free to expensive. Some centers, like the Respite program at the Brookdale Center on Aging in New York City, have no fixed fee; they ask only for a contribution.

The fee generally includes meals and laundry. When you want to drop off your relative in the morning and pick her up in the evening, you pay by the hour. The fee for a whole day, including an overnight stay, is proportionately reduced, so it is not as expensive as counting the total number of hours.

The center I visited cost only $3.00 per hour, $40 for a whole day and overnight stay, and $240 for a week's stay. This is very reasonable, considering that the average cost was $75 to $175 *per day* depending on the region.

Respite care is completely covered by Medicaid for eligible persons, even at the more luxurious centers. There is a sliding scale of fees based on financial need for private-paying guests.

Respite Care at Home

This simply involves having a home-care worker or volunteer supervise the sick person in her own home while you take an extended break. A major advantage of in-home respite care is that Alzheimer's patients, who typically find change unbearable, remain in a familiar environment. Another advantage is that it can quickly be provided during an emergency, such as a caregiver's hospitalization.

Fee-based Home Respite Care

Local social service and health agencies can arrange for a home care worker to come to your home a few hours each day or week. The fee is modest and based on ability to pay.

Some long-term care facilities also provide respite care at home. This has several advantages: (1) Medical therapy, nursing and other health care services are available for dementia victims who have other health problems. (2) It prepares the sick person and the family for eventual permanent institutional care.

A nursing home that has an Alzheimer's emergency respite program can offer round-the-clock care in the patient's home for three to seven days per week. A week's advance notice is advisable, although in some cases a caregiver can get immediate respite care. Family counseling and referrals to other services in the community are also provided. Fees are based on ability to pay.

Volunteer In-home Respite Care

Many caregivers arrange with relatives, friends, and neighbors to come in for a few days at a time when needed.

Thanks to Alzheimer Association chapters, the number of volunteer in-home respite programs is growing. Some are joint endeavors with a community organization or government agency. The chapters screen and recruit people who live in the community. After a brief training on how to care for dementia victims, the volunteers are ready to offer several hours of respite per visit in the homes of overburdened caregivers. They provide companionship and simple recreational activities, but they are not responsible for skilled nursing tasks, housekeeping, bathing or meal preparation. Details of the program vary in each chapter.

The local church, synagogue or temple and senior citizen center may also provide volunteers free of charge..

Several types of simultaneous home care can be arranged. You can enroll your sick relative in a day care center, have home aides come on a prearranged schedule or as needed, place him/her in a respite center whenever you need more time off from your responsibilities, and have volunteers come in occasionally.

NURSING HOMES

Like many caregivers, I resisted placing my mother in a nursing home until a crisis forced me to do so. My resistance was due to misunderstandings and needless fears — the level of care provided would not be as good as the care I was giving; Mom would be miserable and maybe mistreated; family, friends and neighbors would think I was shirking my duty; my traditional belief that it was the family's responsibility; nursing homes are cold, bureaucratic institutions.

I was wrong on all counts. Not only did Mom get good care, she also had an active social life and seemed happier than when she sat home alone all day with only occasional visitors.

I was also surprised to find the nursing home had a friendly community-like atmosphere among the residents, staff and administrators which almost made visiting Mom a pleasant experience. In some ways it almost made up for the social life I had missed since I began taking care of her.

Every situation is different. In my case, caring for Mom by myself, with no family member nearby, it was the appropriate care option when she became incontinent and started wandering at night and getting lost.

However, placing a loved one in a nursing home will not entirely free caregivers of anxiety and worry. Studies show there is little difference in stress symptoms between caregivers who provide 24 hours-a-day care at home and those whose relatives are in a long-term care facility. This is because the caregiver still has a strong commitment to the patient.

Selecting a Nursing Home

Don't wait till the last minute before starting your search for a nursing home. I was lucky in that the decision was made by the hospital social worker. It takes a lot of time to research and visit several places to find the right one. Also, good nursing homes, especially those with Alzheimer units, often have long waiting lists.

Get as much information as you can before making a final choice. Talk with members of an Alzheimer support group. When you visit a nursing home, talk with the staff. Talk with visiting family members. Ask questions.

Make sure the nursing home is covered by Medicaid and by long-term private insurance.

Excellent sources of information for me were the nursing home division of the New York City Department of Aging and a social worker at the hospital where my mother was evaluated and diagnosed.

Also, make sure the nursing home is near enough for family members to visit as often as they like.

Physical Setting

Don't assume that a nursing home with elegant accommodations and/or a high price provides better care than a modest one. The quality of relationships that exist among staff members, residents and their relatives makes a crucial difference.

The hallways in Mom's nursing home are painted in soft peach, a cheerful and soothing color, and the residents' rooms have a homey look with attractive wallpaper and curtains. Residents can furnish their rooms with their own television or radio sets, photographs and small decorative items. Each room has a spanking clean bathroom with a safety bar. The lighting is bright enough to uplift one's spirits but without the glare that can be harmful to a confused dementia resident.

Hallways and residents' rooms are free of clutter.

There is a common room on each floor that is also used as a dining room. On the main floor there is a large reception room where recreational activities, birthday parties, and special events take place. Ambulatory residents use it when they don't want to stay in their rooms. Adjoining the main reception room is an outside patio.

Health conditions in nursing homes are periodically inspected by the state or federal government. A *certificate of inspection* is posted or made available to visitors.

A copy of *Resident's Rights* is posted near an entrance.

Size and Population

Some professionals believe dementia patients function better in small units of eight to fifteen people each, but this can be expensive for families. Nevertheless, many nursing homes offer good care in larger units.

Quality of Care

There are no strong urine odors. The residents are clean and show no untreated skin sores or other afflictions. Mom's dermatitis, which used to drive me crazy, cleared up significantly in the nursing home.

Qualified professionals with geriatric training are available: physician, nurse, physical therapist, dentist, dietician, etc. They visit the residents regularly and are available for consultation. There also is a beauty parlor in the building.

Medications to keep residents quiet and under control are never administered without the written consent of a family member.

Activities

Posted by the elevator on each floor are lists and charts that help orient the residents and give visitors a glimpse of life in the home: a calendar of morning, afternoon, and evening activities scheduled for the week printed in large letters; a chart of daily menus for the week; in the common room of each unit, a large chart with special activities for the day printed in large letters — television, music, song fests, dances, bingo, physical exercise, word games, blackboard games, art class, music & dancing, story time, movies, exercise games, spelling bee.

Residents are not treated as passive puppets. They are encouraged to do as much for themselves as their abilities allow, such as personal care and light housekeeping. One of Mom's "buddies," little old lady in a wheelchair, would proudly recite to me, in excruciating detail, how neatly she kept her room. I had to listen to this each time I visited Mom.

Staff

The mood of the staff is reflected on the general atmosphere and greatly influences the residents. In Mom's nursing home they generally seem friendly, cheerful and satisfied in their jobs.

Staff members receive continuing education in patient care.

On each floor, the staff remains relatively stable. Dementia victims need the security of having familiar persons around.

According to the experts, a large staff does not guarantee good care. However, a staff shortage can make those who are present tense and irritable and causes them to rush the residents.

Most of the residents appear comfortable and some even seem happy. Those who look angry or tense are in the late stage of dementia. In fact, Mom seems less anxious and fearful than when she lived at home. Whenever I bring her over for a visit, she soon wants to "go back home."

Most of the staff members do not talk down to the residents. They treat them as adults and with affection and dignity. When I took Mom to visit her old neighbors on the fourth floor, staff members rushed up to greet her by name and seemed genuinely happy to see her.

Other residents on the floor are at the same level of functioning as your relative. According to some professionals, residents who are in the later stages of dementia should be apart from others. However, some facilities have successfully mixed people who are at different stages of dementia.

Cost

High fees, like a flashy environment, do not guarantee quality care. The cost of nursing home care is so high that even middle income people cannot afford it. (In 1992, yearly nursing home fees in New York City averaged about $75,000.) To avoid losing the family's life savings, many people see an Elder Law attorney for advice on their eligibility for public entitlement programs and the legal transfer of assets and property.

Avoid a Facility That:

Views its main function as restraining and protecting residents rather than stimulating their remaining capacities.

Treats residents like children or imbeciles.

Has "activity" programs consisting solely or mainly of sitting idle or watching TV. Unless your loved one has an advanced stage of dementia, avoid a facility that only provides custodial care to residents.

Claims it can postpone or prevent the decline of dementia or restore mental abilities. Such a facility should be immediately reported to the local Alzheimer's Association chapter and the Department of Aging.

Is a Special Unit Right for Your Loved One?

A new trend in nursing home care is to include a special unit for dementia victims. These are called Dedicated Dementia Care Units or Special Care Units. Most of them are privately owned and operated.

The physical setting, recreation, and social activities are all regarded as aspects of therapy, and are designed to keep residents functioning at their highest cognitive level as long as possible. The following is a summary of information from several special care units that you may find useful.

The results can be astonishing, as shown in the following excerpts from a newspaper report on the Grace Plaza Heritage Unit located in Great Neck, NY:[5] *It has restored life to many ... patients. They're now able to talk about events that were integral to their past, to relate to things that had meaning to them before (losing) their formidable resources .... Residents who had been withdrawn, anxious, aggressive and dependent show increases in socialization, appetite and independent activities, and a decrease in agitation and wandering .... They are calmer and happier.*

Physical Setting

Visual, tactile and auditory stimuli are selected which stimulate memories of the past; e.g., paintings and murals depicting typical outdoor scenes and activities of the community's former days; a barbershop with a striped pole; movie theater posters of old-time movie stars; a photograph of each resident as a young person on the bedroom door; "theme" walls that display mementoes of love, marriage, and family life; a living room with the comfortable look of the residents' own homes and furnishings.

Activities

There is a music and arts center that provides old movies; group singing of old familiar songs; sports, games, and crafts from the past; a cheerful kitchenette where residents can engage in familiar activities under supervision, like mixing batter and kneading dough, making salads, watering the plants; fashion shows featuring clothing from a past era; weekly visits of animals from nearby shelters; copies of old Jack Benny and Al Jolson radio shows; popular old dances like lindy, waltz and fox trot; gardening.

---

[5]Reprinted with permission "Is Familiar Milieu an Alzheimer Rx? New York Times 5/17/92

Caution: Charging a high fee or segregating residents according to their level of functioning does not make a program special. Some programs claim they are "special" when they only provide the good care all residents should receive.

Where to Go For Information and Help

- The local Alzheimer Association chapter has information on nursing homes in your area. It can give you checklists that will help you select a good nursing home. See also the checklist in *The 36-Hour Day* by Nancy Mace & Peter Rabins and other sources listed in the Appendix E.

- Many Area Agencies on Aging give free information and help with placement.

- The local Department for the Aging may have a residential and nursing home affairs unit that offers information and counseling. It may also help caregivers evaluate the nursing home needs of relatives and level of care required, and recommend an appropriate facility.

- Local Department of Social Services, Division of Adult Services.

- You may also wish to contact state or national associations of nursing homes. See Appendix E for names and addresses.

ADULT HOMES

These are long-term care facilities that admit frail elderly persons and mentally impaired younger persons. Some also admit people who have early or middle stage dementia. Some adult homes serve members of a particular ethnic or religious affiliation.

Services

These usually include room and board, supervised activities and outings, housekeeping, and some personal care (help with bathing and dressing). Nursing or medical services are not provided, but some homes contract with physicians who visit residents when necessary. Since they are not licensed or inspected as often as nursing homes, visit often to make sure your relative continues receiving quality care.

Admission

Only persons who are ambulatory are accepted. Clients who are incontinent and/or wander are not admitted.

Cost

In 1993, the average rate for a shared room in New York City was $1,200 a month and private room rates were between $1,700 and $2,000 a month. Elsewhere, the cost would be lower.

Many adult homes accept Social Security, Supplemental Security Income, or Social Security Disability if a concerned person will make up the difference between the government check and the private pay rate.

Caution: A few homes have admitted persons who can pay privately and then tried to evict them when their assets were depleted.

What to Look for in an Adult Home

Look into the following criteria, *which also apply to nursing homes and respite centers*:

Is it near enough so family and friends can visit regularly?

Cleanliness: Are hallways free of clutter that could be a special safety hazard to an Alzheimer's victim?

Security: Is someone on watch 24 hours a day?

How do staff members relate to residents? Are they friendly, respectful or are they angry and patronizing?

Is there a program of planned activities?

Will frail, elderly persons with Alzheimer's disease be safe and comfortable with much younger, mentally impaired residents?

FINDING CARE FOR SOMEONE WHO LIVES FAR AWAY

What can you do to help a loved one who has dementia and lives alone? How do you get information about eligibility requirements for services in another city or state? How do you know what kinds of services s/he needs? How can you arrange for medical and home care without getting into an airplane and staying over for months of fact finding and dealing with bureaucratic red tape and a maze of social agencies? The following can help you:

Contact the Alzheimer's Association and the Area Agency on Aging in that community. They will put you in touch with groups that provide in-home care, nursing, emergency services, Meal-on-Wheels, transportation, legal assistance and adult day care. However, you still have to do the research and paperwork, and oversee the quality of care given to your relative. This can take many months of your time.

For a Fee, Geriatric Care Consultants Will:

- Assess what kind of care your relative needs.
- Decide the most effective and least expensive care plan.

- Arrange for and monitor home aide and home health care.
- Arrange for nursing home placement when needed.
- Arrange for delivery of hot meals.
- Determine your relative's eligibility for financial aid.
- Do the paperwork and research involved.
- Provide crisis intervention, individual and family counseling, and bereavement counseling.

Cost

The average initial consulting fee is about $150. A complete assessment may cost about $300. Once care is provided for, the consultant's services might be needed for an hour every few weeks at an hourly rate of from $30 to $85.

For Names of Consultants Who Live in or near Your Sick Relative, Contact:

- National Association of Private Geriatric Care Managers, 655 North Alveron Way, Tucson, AZ 85711 ☎ (602) 881-8008. Many of them are experienced social workers and registered nurses.
- Aging Network Services, 4400 East-West Highway, Ste 907, Bethesda, MD 20814. This is a for-profit network of social workers.
- Look in the Yellow Pages under "Geriatric ----" or "Older Care ----."

Check the Reputation and Experience of a Consultant.

As there are no state certifications for this new profession, you must rely on your own investigation. You can get detailed information on how to evaluate the qualifications of a geriatric care consultant from the National Association of Private Geriatric Care Managers (see above) and *Beat the Nursing Home Trap* by Joseph Matthews (Nolo Press, Berkeley. 1994).

If you can't afford a private consultant, call the Eldercare Locator (800) 677-1116. This toll-free, nationwide information and referral service will give you information on local agencies that provide adult day care, meal delivery, legal services, transportation and more. It's sponsored by the US Administration on Aging.

Public and non-profit social service agencies also offer many of the same services.

Appendix D

LEGAL AND FINANCIAL INFORMATION YOU MAY NEED

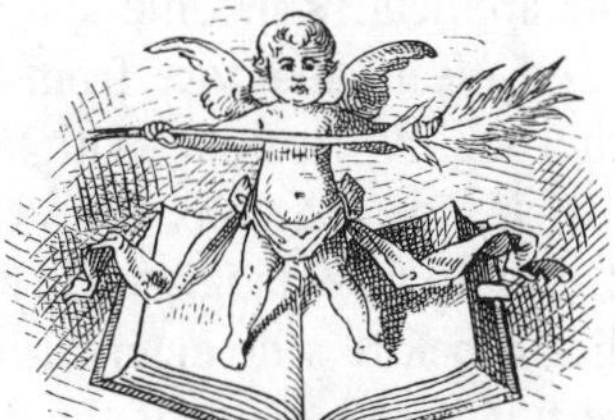

NOTE:

The following information is a general guide only. It is not intended to provide legal advice that applies to any specific situation. Readers are advised to consult with professionals who are up-to-date on changes in federal and state laws regarding financial aid to sick and elderly persons. Before applying for Medicaid and nursing home admission, it is advisable to consult an expert on elder law, especially if there are special circumstances relating to the applicant's income and assets.

Do not rely on well-meaning advice from family and friends who may not be thoroughly familiar with the law and your special circumstances. If, for example, following such advice a house is transferred to a son or daughter, it may disqualify the applicant from Medicaid before s/he enters a nursing home or it may impose a severe financial penalty if the person has already been admitted to a nursing home.

The costs of long-term care can be ruinous. As soon as you have a medical diagnosis of dementia (even before, if it is suspected), get as much information as possible on the various types of public benefit and entitlement programs (including Medicaid) that your loved one might be eligible to receive. Learn about the laws regarding incompetency, wills, and surrogate decision-making. Consult an elder law attorney about legal ways of sheltering assets and transferring property.

This section summarizes the major legal and financial matters you should know about. It gives an overview of the types of help that are available at this time and what you need to do regarding legal and financial aspects of long-term care. It also directs you to additional sources of help and information you may need. Medicare and most private health insurance plans did not cover long term health care in the home or institution as this book was going to press. Many long-term care insurance plans provided limited benefits and excluded home care and preexisting conditions.

The situation is not entirely bleak, however. Like many caregivers, you and/or your loved one may be eligible for financial assistance from federal, state, country, or local sources without realizing it. However, be prepared to dig long and hard to get it. You may even be tempted to give up in frustration — more than once, as I did — before your attempts pay off. The problem does not lie in you. The rules regarding benefit eligibility and financing are so complex and change so often that even the experts find it difficult to keep up.

GETTING STARTED

FIRST, you'll need proof of your relative's disability in order to apply for financial assistance as well as disability benefits from his/her employer or from the Social Security administration. Without such proof the family's health insurance coverage under his plan, or support for any dependent children still living at home, may also be at risk.

NEXT, start learning about the legal and financial aspects of long-term care. Plan as far ahead as possible so you can avoid delays in receiving the benefits and services your loved one will eventually need. A delay could cost you money, even your home!

If your sick relative is still able to understand the issues involved and make his/her wishes known, he should also take part in the legal and financial planning.

FINANCIAL AND HEALTH CARE BENEFITS YOU SHOULD KNOW ABOUT

The cost of nursing home care and long-term care at home is so high that few families can afford it without plunging into poverty. Recently, some insurance companies have made long-term care insurance available, but this is of little benefit to those who already have the illness.

If the thought of receiving government financial aid and health care benefits bothers you, as it did me, stop and think how many years you and your loved one have paid taxes into it. These entitlements were created as a kind of national insurance to help citizens who are down on their luck. It hurts, but believe me, you'll get used to it.

There are two kinds of assistance your sick relative may be eligible to receive: (1) Those that provide income for the sick person and/or dependent family members, (2) Those that help pay for medical expenses, including nursing home care.

Medicare and Medicaid are the two government programs that help pay medical costs. As I am writing this, high-level discussions were taking place on ways to change the laws to give medical protection to all citizens.

Medicare

This is a federal health insurance program for people age sixty-five or older who are receiving Social Security retirement benefits. A person with Alzheimer's disease who is younger than sixty-five must receive Social Security Disability benefits for 24 months before becoming eligible to receive Medicare.

It helps pay for inpatient hospital care and limited skilled nursing care while recuperating from an illness. It also covers part of the cost of doctors' fees and other medical items.

It does **NOT**, however, pay for nursing home care, and it may cover less than 50% of the cost of other medical services unless the physician or other provider accepts Medicare "assignment." This means they will accept the Medicare rate for the services provided and not bill the patient for more. Families who care for an Alzheimer's victim are not helped much by this program.

Medicaid

This is a joint federal/state program that provides medical care to the needy. The laws and regulations governing the program are mind boggling and constantly changing. The following is a brief summary of major points that are important to family caregivers. For more information on eligibility criteria and application procedures, contact the sources listed below.

The federal government sets minimum standards that all state Medicaid programs must meet. Beyond that, each state decides how much its programs will cover. For example, all state plans must cover nursing home costs. But each state sets its own eligibility standards for deciding who is "medically needy" (people who cannot pay for their medical care, but who are not otherwise destitute). Consultation, preferably with an elder law attorney who knows the special conditions concerning your state, is advisable to protect the family's income and assets.

Medicaid Offers More Comprehensive Health Coverage than Medicare

It includes adult day care, long-term nursing home care, and full-time home care for Alzheimer's patients. It is the major source of funding to protect families from becoming impoverished because of a chronic or catastrophic illness.

The level of protection also varies from state to state. It can cover all or part of nursing home costs. Some states provide no help at all, even to families near the poverty level, as many caregivers learn to their horror.

Despite the strict eligibility rules, most people in nursing homes are on Medicaid, and many of them are classified as "middle-income." They and their relatives consulted with experts on spousal protection rules and the legal transfer of assets before it was too late.

Eligibility Criteria for Medicaid

Eligibility is determined by income, assets, and financial need. Usually, Medicaid is available only to applicants whose assets and income fall below the federal poverty level. However, there are special conditions that protect the spouse or adult child caregiver from impoverishment.

Persons who are ***not*** residing in a nursing home must meet the following federal guidelines on limits to the amount of income and assets they are allowed to keep and still be eligible for Medicaid. The figures vary in each state and you should find out what these are in your state.

The assets and income of children and other relatives are not counted, even if they live with the applicant.

If the applicant lives with his/her spouse, both their income and assets are counted. But if they are divorced or legally separated and living apart, only the applicant's income and assets, plus any financial support from the other spouse, are counted.

Monthly Income: The single applicant (the sick person) is allowed a maximum monthly income of about $300 to $500; a couple, about $500 to $700. All sources of income are counted — government benefits, including Social Security, employment income, rent, interest or dividends from savings and investments, pensions, annuities, gifts and royalties. A spouse who is employed is allowed to keep the first $65 per month plus one-half of the amount over that. The total maximum limits vary according to family size. Also, under the surplus income program, there are certain exceptions that allow a person to be eligible.

Assets: A person who is not residing in a nursing home is allowed a maximum of $2000 in non-exempt assets; ($3000) for a couple. Some types and amounts of assets are exempt; e.g., a burial fund of $1,500, up to $2000 worth of household and personal items, a car not exceeding a value of $4,500, the applicant's home if s/he or the spouse is still living in it. In some states, the spouse is allowed additional protected assets as high as $66,480.

Special Rules Apply to Nursing Home Residents

Medicaid pays almost all nursing home costs for a resident who meets eligibility requirements.

Income

In about 19 states, a single resident whose monthly income exceeds the limit of from about $700 to $1,100 does not qualify for Medicaid coverage. The other states have no income limits in order to be eligible, but almost all of the resident's income goes to the nursing home to reduce the amount Medicaid pays.

The rules for married couples living together differ. In most states, income received in the name of the spouse living at home is not counted towards the state's maximum limit. If more than half their joint income is in the name of the nursing home resident, the spouse living at home is allowed to keep about $750 to $1,500 of that income as a living allowance. The limits vary in each state.

Assets

Single nursing home residents whose assets exceed the following limits will be eligible for Medicaid only after they pay for their nursing homes costs until the limits are reached. Medicaid refers to this as "spending down." The following figures may vary in your state.

- maximum of $2000 in savings, stocks or certificates of deposit.
- car not exceeding $4,500 in value.
- up to $1,500 for burial expenses and a burial plot.
- household and personal items not exceeding $2000 in value.
- life insurance policy not exceeding $1,500 in value.
- place of residence

Limits to the combined assets of married residents whose spouses live at home vary from state to state, but generally they are as follows:

- place of residence, regardless of value.
- one car, regardless of value.
- furniture and household items, regardless of value.
- life insurance not exceeding a face value of $1,500.
- two burial plots and up to $1,500 per person for burial costs.

▸ up to $6000 of items required for maintaining the place of residence

▸ one-half the value of all other assets owned at the time the sick person enters the nursing home.

Transfer of Assets

There are rules regarding the legal transfer of assets and income in order to qualify for Medicaid. The rules are strict to prevent the transfer of excess assets.

In some cases, a person can transfer assets on one day and qualify for *home care benefits* on the very next day. *This does not apply to nursing home care.* There is a waiting period, called a "lookback" period, before a Medicaid application is filed or the applicant enters a nursing home.

Transfers made *before* the look-back period will not affect eligibility, whatever the size of the transfer, the motive for the transfer, or the transferee.

But transfers made *during* the look-back period are considered invalid unless they fall into a permitted category. (See below.) This will not disqualify you for Medicaid but will delay payment of benefits for a period of time calculated by dividing the value of the assets transferred by the average monthly cost of nursing home care in the area. These are usually so high that few applicants must wait out the full period (unless the transfer is very large or the state has unusually low costs). Originally, the look-back period in all states was 30 months or 24 months, depending on nursing home costs in the community. New legislation is expected to increase the lookback period to 36 months or impose no limitation on the ineligibility period.

Allowable Transfers

Transfer of title to the home can be made to the following:

Applicant's spouse.

Minor child or a blind or disabled child of any age.

Child of any age who has lived in the home and taken care of the applicant for a minimum of two years prior to his/her entry to a nursing home.

Sibling, if the sibling had an equity interest in the home before the transfer, and lived with the applicant for at least one year prior to his/her entry to a nursing home.

Additional exemptions include transfer of a car worth up to $4,500, personal and household items worth up to $2000, and other assets.

Of all allowable exemptions, transfer of the home to the spouse receives the most protection. There is no requirement that the spouse have had a prior equity interest or provided care. The transfer is also free of gift and estate tax. The state Medicaid agency cannot put a lien on the house, or recover the cost of custodial care, while the spouse (or minor or disabled child or adult child caregiver) is still living in the home.

How to Apply for Medicaid

▸ Get a Disability Documentation Kit from your local Alzheimer's Association chapter or write to its national organization. It tells what records you'll need in order to prove eligibility.

▸ Have a P.R.I. (Patient Review Instrument) and a Screen form completed by a professional certified by the Department of Health. This form assesses the level of care your sick relative needs. The way it is completed is very important in deciding eligibility. The medical center where the diagnosis was made, the Department for the Aging, or other agencies will direct you to a nurse qualified to complete the form. The family caregiver (or anyone else who spends the most time with the sick person) should be present when it is being completed.

▸ If you have been living in your parent's home during the look-back period and have taken care of her, you'll have to prove it. Collect as much evidence as you can: letters; credit card statements; bank books; tax records; house bills that you've paid such as repairs, mortgage, utilities, furnishings, etc. Don't be surprised if all your evidence fills a small suitcase. The more, the better. **Do not send originals.**

▸ *Make photocopies of important documents* concerning the applicant, spouse (even though deceased), and adult child caregiver, like:

Birth and death certificates

Cemetery plot deed

Stock and bond certificates

Bank statements

Medicare and Social Security cards

Copies of bills and credit card statements that prove you have paid for at least some home expenses

Also *make copies of every form you complete and every letter you write* regarding the application. This will make it easier to appeal should your application be denied. Many applications are initially rejected, but are approved when the rejection is appealed. (See fair hearing below.)

Also *keep a log of every person you talk to* (name, date, time, advice given). I decided to do this after learning that some so-called experts gave me conflicting advice! Moreover, a review of my notes later helped me understand the very complex eligibility rules.

FINANCIAL SUPPORT PROGRAMS

Social Security Disability

These are payments to wage earners under age 65 who can no longer work because they are disabled. There must be proof, in the form of medical statements and other documentation, of inability to work. The definition, "functional disability," now includes Alzheimer's disease.

Monthly payments are based on the person's past earnings. The applicant must have worked a minimum of five of the past ten years, but the years do not have to be consecutive.

To apply, contact your local Social Security office. Don't be surprised if your application is rejected. Many applicants are at first. There is an appeal process, and many persons who were initially denied eventually receive benefits.

Supplemental Security Income (SSI)

This program guarantees a minimum monthly income to persons who have limited income and assets and are 65 or older, disabled, or blind. It's important to apply immediately after you get a diagnosis of Alzheimer's disease because payments begin with the date of application or date of eligibility.

To qualify as a disabled person, an Alzheimer's (or other related dementia) victim must have proof that s/he is unemployable.

However, if the applicant is also over sixty-five, she may get higher payment by qualifying as an "aged" person rather than disabled.

Applicants are allowed to have some financial or property assets, including a small amount of cash, a home, and modest income, and still qualify for SSI. However, SSI payments are reduced by outside income.

In most states, a person eligible for SSI is also eligible for Medicaid, other social services, and disability benefits provided by the state or county.

General Public Assistance

This program helps persons who do not qualify for Social Security disability, supplemental security income or other benefit programs. Since eligibility requirements are strict and payments are low — less than $100 a month, sometimes for a period as brief as three months — it should be regarded as a temporary source of money while waiting for confirmation of Social Security or SSI eligibility or for the first check.

Veterans Administration Benefits

This is for veterans who need hospitalization, respite care or nursing home care. Contact the VA General Information Office (810 Vermont Avenue, NW, Washington, D.C. 20420 ☎ 202/233-4000) or a local VA office.

Other Programs to Assist Elderly Persons

While some are for low income persons, the **Older Americans Act (OAA) programs** are available to all persons 60 years of age or older. The services include Visiting Nurses, Meals on Wheels, and home repair. These are available through the local Area Agency on Aging, senior centers, social service agencies, and religious organizations.

Fair Hearings

If your application for Medicaid assistance or entitlements such as Disability benefits is rejected, or if you believe the benefit funds granted are too little or terminated, you can appeal by requesting a fair hearing.

If you appeal a Medicaid decision, it's best to have an attorney advise and be with you at the hearing.

LEGAL MATTERS YOU SHOULD KNOW ABOUT

Get Expert Advice

It's important to understand thoroughly the issues involved before you apply for public entitlements and benefits, especially Medicaid. Do this as soon as you have a diagnosis of dementia. Don't wait until long-term institutional or home care becomes necessary. The expenses can be ruinous.

You may not need to consult an attorney. Whether or not you do depends on how you feel about the following:

- Your sick relative has enough income or assets to pay for nursing home care and you need advice on how best to manage these resources.
- You are confused by some issues and how the eligibility rules apply to your situation.
- The laws regarding eligibility for Medicaid are constantly changing and there are many exceptions that allow for unique family situations. Yours may be one.

- To protect the family from becoming impoverished, to prevent losing the family home, you need to know how to legally transfer assets.

- The language of the regulations is full of contradictions. You might be able to understand it if you have the time, patience, and a head for slogging through voluminous pages of legalese.

Not all lawyers have experience with elder law, specifically laws concerning Alzheimer's and related dementias, trusts, estates, and Medicare and Medicaid provisions. So, find an expert who keeps up-to-date on the rapidly changing situation. It shouldn't be difficult because more attorneys are specializing in elder law.

Elder law specialists can also help with estate planning, wills, powers of attorney, and other legal matters. They will also advise and represent you if your application is rejected and you request a fair hearing.

Durable Power of Attorney

This allows the sick person to designate someone, not necessarily a relative, to act legally on her behalf when she can no longer manage her financial, legal and/or personal affairs. The power granted can cover everything or be limited to certain assets or activities such as paying bills and writing checks. It can become effective as soon as the document is signed and continue to operate after the person becomes incapacitated, or it can go into effect only upon incapacity. The lawyer usually prepares the document which you must then have notarized. Stationery stores that stock legal documents also have the forms.

At the time the document is signed, the sick person must be able to understand the powers being conveyed. It may not be too late for persons in the early to moderate stages of dementia to make their wishes known, as long as the document is signed during a period of lucidity.

Now you know why it's important to deal with the legal and financial issues as soon as possible. Don't allow your depression or denial to put things off until the last minute.

A Power of Attorney that is not durable gives the agent authority to act on the patient's behalf any time **before** the patient becomes incapacitated, but not after.

Living Trust

This allows a person (the grantor) to place his assets in a trust and appoint a relative or trusted friend (the trustee) to manage some or all of them. The assets must be managed according to the terms of the trust and for the benefit of the grantor. The arrangement is revocable, allowing the grantor to make changes if he wishes. Also, he can serve as trustee while he is capable of making competent decisions. After that, the trustee appointed by him takes over.

A major reason for obtaining a living trust is to avoid the high legal costs and time involved in probate, whereby the court supervises the distribution of the estate.

Living Will

This stipulates which health care decisions, such as life support, are (or are not) to be carried out should the person become mentally incapacitated.

Health Care Proxy

This is a power of attorney that allows a person to appoint someone else to make treatment decisions on her behalf when she no longer has the capacity to do so. It's available in many states, but not all.

A lawyer is not needed to prepare a living will and health care proxy. You can get forms from the Alzheimer's Association, fill them out and have them witnessed and signed, then notarized. Be aware that some states restrict the validity of a health care proxy to that state.

Transfer of Title to Property

The term "property" refers to items like real estate, bank deposits, and stock certificates. Transfer of title to some or all these can be made to a spouse, family member or a friend.

It's advisable to consult with an elder law attorney on how to legally transfer the sick person's property, including those that are jointly-owned, and to do so *long before* the need for long-term care arrives. There is a "look back" waiting period (see above) which varies from state to state.

Moreover, the tax, public benefits, and other legal issues involved are too complex for many of us to understand.

Conservatorship of Property

This is a legal document that protects a person's interests **after** she is no longer competent to make decisions concerning her future. It is usually not necessary if a durable power of attorney has been signed. A petition to establish a conservatorship can be filed by a relative, friend, or other interested party. Otherwise, the court will appoint a conservator to care for the person's property when she becomes incapacitated, and the court will supervise the conservator's management of the sick person's assets to ensure that her needs are met.

Guardianship

This operates in the same manner as a conservatorship of property. When the person can no longer care for his personal needs, a guardian is appointed by the court. The guardian has full responsibility for his physical care and welfare, and has the power to place him in a nursing home if he can no longer be cared for at home.

Representative Payee

This is an arrangement whereby a person who is incapable of managing her public benefits (Social Security, Veterans, etc.) can have a third party appointed to receive the benefit checks, cash them and manage the proceeds.

How to Consult with an Attorney

The better prepared you are before hiring an elder law attorney, the less it will cost in time and money, In 1993, a private attorney cost between $100 and $200 an hour. Write down specifically what you want regarding legal and financial matters and what questions to ask **before** you make an appointment.

When you arrive for an appointment, come prepared with photocopies of documents and written details concerning the sick person:

Bank accounts

Birth certificate

Death certificate or divorce papers of the spouse, if the sick person is widowed or divorced

Deeds for property owned by the sick person

Documents (including dates) regarding transfers of assets and/or gifts

Income, including pension and social security

Insurance policies

Investments

Loans

Mortgages

Tax returns

Written will or other written wishes of the sick person

If you are a spouse, an adult child caregiver, or a disabled child living in the home, also bring documents that prove you meet the requirements for the exceptions discussed above.

Also come prepared with a list of written questions you want to ask. You will be given so much information during the first hour that it's best to take notes, so bring a notebook and pen too. Do not bring a tape recorder unless you are given persmission to do so by the attorney.

Where to Get Expert Legal Help

Alzheimer's Association chapters can give you information on legal resources in your area and names of attorneys who have experience in legal matters regarding Alzheimer's disease. They also offer free or low cost literature and sponsor seminars and workshops on legal and financial matters. Some chapters also help Alzheimer patients and their families with legal and financial planning.

Other sources of elder law attorneys include the nearest law school, the state bar association, and the local Bar Association.

Personal references are an excellent source of finding professionals. Speak to your friends, family, and Alzheimer support group members.

Send for a list of elder law attorneys in your area by writing to: National Academy of Elder Law Attorneys, 1730 East River Road, Ste. 107, Tucson, AZ 85718. Include a stamped, self-addressed envelope.

Area Agencies on Aging offer information on public benefits. They may also sponsor free legal services for the indigent elderly. Write to the National Association of Area Agencies on Aging, 1112 16th Street NW, Ste. 100, Washington, D.C. 20036 ☏ (202) 296-8130.

Community social service agencies and senior centers offer information on public benefit programs. They will also help you fill out complicated application forms. It was a local social service agency that started me on the long road that eventually ended with finding a good nursing home and obtaining Medicaid eligibility for Mom.

Appendix E

WHERE TO GO FOR MORE INFORMATION

Books, newspaper and magazine articles, government reports and scientific journals on Alzheimer's disease can be found in your local library, senior centers, and mental health centers. Lending libraries are also available in adult day care centers, respite centers and nursing homes.

City, County and State Agencies on Aging also distribute helpful information. The New York State Office for the Aging, for example, offers the following free literature: *Caring: Helping Your Elderly Spouse or Family Member; Coping with Alzheimer's Disease; Senior Handbook* (lists addresses and phone numbers for aging resources).

Your local Department for the Aging may offer a guide like *Alzheimer's Disease: Where To Go For Help In New York City* which is distributed by the Alzheimer's Resource Center, New York City Department for the Aging. This free directory includes information on diagnostic centers, adult day care, home care, support groups, residential and in-home respite programs, how to care for an Alzheimer's patient at home, and where to go for financial and legal counseling and help in nursing home placement. A similar directory of resources in your local area can be obtained from your Alzheimer's association chapter.

Alzheimer Association Chapters have a lending library and offer free or low cost materials, some of which are listed below. You can also get information from the Benjamin B. Green Field library at the Association's headquarters in Chicago. It's a multi-media resource center that has almost every kind of data relating to Alzheimer's disease, including videotapes, children's books and bibliographies. If you have a modem and personal computer, the data can be accessed directly ☎ (312) 335 9602.

ADULT DAY CARE

Alzheimer's Day Care: A Basic Guide, by Lindeman, David A., *et. al.* New York: Hemisphere Publishing Corporation.

National Directory of Adult Day Care Centers. Your local library may have a copy of this 449-page directory of over 2,000 adult day care centers. To order send $149 + $6 shipping to Human Resources Publishing 3100 Highway 138; Wall Township, NJ 07719-1442.

Why Adult Day Care? Free from the National Institute on Adult Day Care, 600 Maryland Avenue SW, West Wing 100, Washington, D.C. 20024.

ALZHEIMER'S DISEASE AND RELATED DEMENTIAS

The following free and low cost materials are available from the Alzheimer's Association:

Alzheimer's Disease: A Description Of The Dementias (free)

Alzheimer's Disease: An Overview (free)

Aronson, Miriam K., Ed.D., ed. *Understanding Alzheimer's Disease*. Charles Scribner's Sons. ($15.95)

Clinical Diagnosis of Alzheimer's Disease (free)

Differential Diagnosis of Alzheimer's Disease (free)

Fact Sheet on Alzheimer's Disease (free)

If You Think Someone You Know Has Alzheimer's Disease (free)

If You Have Alzheimer's Disease (free)

Memory and Aging ($0.85.)

Steps to Choosing a Physician

The Vanishing Mind: a Practical Guide to Alzheimer's Disease and Related Illnesses. by Heston, White, Freeman & Co, 1991. ($15.95)

The Younger Alzheimer's Patient

HOME CARE

Carroll, David. *When Your Loved One Has Alzheimer's: A Caregiver's Guide Based on Methods Developed by The Brookdale Center on Aging*. New York: Harper and Row.

Confused Minds, Burdened Families: Finding Help for People with Alzheimer's and Other Dementias, # OTA-BA-403, Supt. of Documents, U.S. Government Printing Office, Washington, D.C. 20402.

Couper, Donna. *Aging and Our Families: Handbook for Family Caregivers.* Human Sciences Press, Inc.

Foster, Phyllis, ed. *Therapeutic Activities With the Impaired Elderly.* The Haworth Press, NY.

Gruetzner, Howard. *Alzheimer's: A Caregiver's Guide and Source Book*. John Wiley and Sons.

McGuire, Francis A., et. al., *Therapeutic Humor With the Elderly*. The Haworth Press, NY.

Portnow, M.D., et. al., *Home Care for the Elderly: A Complete Guide.* McGraw-Hill.

Sheridan, Carmel. *Failure Free Activities For The Alzheimer's Patient: A Guidebook for Caregivers*. Cottage Books.

Zgola, V., *Doing Thomeings, A Guide to Programs and Organized Activities for Persons withome Alzheimer's Disease and Related Disorders,* Baltimore, Johns Hopkins University Press.

The following are available from the Alzheimer's Association

Communicating With The Alzheimer's Patient (free)

Especially For The Alzheimer Caregiver (free)

Guide to Home Safety For Caregivers of Persons With Alzheimer's Disease (free)

Home Care With The Alzheimer Patient. $0.95

Just The Facts. This packet contains 15 fact sheets on a variety of topics (eating problems, wandering, incontinence, personal hygiene. $3.00.

Mace, Nancy and P. Rabins. *The Thirty-Six Hour Day.* Baltimore and London: Johns Hopkins University Press. $9.95.

Nassif, Janet Z. *The Home Health Care Solution*. Harper & Row.

Olsen, Richard V. *Homes That Help: Advice From Caregivers for Creating a Supportive Home*. Ideas on how to make the home environment calm, safe and comfortable. Send $13 to NJIT Architecture and Building Science Research Group, University Heights, Newark, NJ 07102.

Personal Health, Guidance In The Care of Patients With Alzheimer's Disease, $0.75.

Steps to Finding Home Care

Steps to Selecting Activities For Persons With Alzheimer's Disease, $1.50.

When The Diagnosis Is Alzheimer's (free)

The following can be ordered from the American Association of Retired Persons. Send title and stock number to AARP, Fulfillment Section, 1909 K Street, NW, Washington, D.C. 20049.

Caregiving. $9.95

Coping and Caring: A Guide for Families with Alzheimer's Patients. #D12441 (free)

Handbook About Care in the Home. #D955 (free)

Miles Away and Still Caring: A Guide for Long-Distance Caregivers. #D12748 (free)

The Gadget Book. $10.95 (AARP members $7.95)

The ***Brookdale Center on Aging*** at Hunter College has the following for professional caregivers. Address: 425 East 25th Street, New York, NY 10010; Attn: Publications. ☏ 212/481-4350.

Home Health Aide Training Manuals. Includes activities, understanding confusion in the client, memory loss and paranoia, verbal and physical abusiveness, encouraging independence and mastery, reminiscence and storytelling, depression and dependency. $24.95; Order # TML-003.

Introduction to Behavior Therapy Terms and Techniques. How to assess and intervene appropriately with difficult behaviors like physical and verbal abuse, wandering, screaming and withdrawal. $49.95; Order # TML-004.

Tapes

Living with Alzheimer's: Your New Video Survival Kit. A three-part video series for caregivers. Information on coping comes from experts in medicine, research, and caregiving. Send

$35 + $4.95 shipping and handling to Long Island Alzheimer's Foundation, 382 Main Street, Port Washington, NY 11050 ☎ (516) 767-9446 to pay by Master Card or Visa.

LEGAL AND FINANCIAL MATTERS

Tomorrow's Choices: preparing Now for Future Legal, Financial, and Health Care Decisions. #D13479. Free from **AARP Fulfillment Section**, 1909 K Street, NW, Washington, D.C. 20049.

Questions & Answers When Looking for an Elder Law Attorney. Free from the National Academy of Elder Law Attorneys, Inc., 655 N Alvernon Way, Ste. 108, Tucson, AZ 85711.

The following free materials are available from your local Alzheimer's Association chapter:

Alzheimer's Disease: A Legal and Financial Planning Guide

Disability Documentation Kit

Financial and Health Care Benefits

Financial Services You May Need

Legal Considerations for Alzheimer's Disease

The following guides are published by the New York State Office for the Aging, Empire State Plaza, Agency Building #2, Albany, NY 12223 ☎ (518) 474-4425. They are are listed here to show what may be available to residents of other states.

Directory of Legal Services for The Elderly

Medicaid for The Elderly, Blind and Disabled in New York State. Overview of federal and New York State laws, benefits and eligibility criteria, application and documentation requirements, rights and responsibilities of beneficiaries, appeals procedures. Send $7.00 and include the order number: PAT-001.

NURSING HOMES

The Nursing Home Handbook. $9.95 (AARP members $6.95). To order write: AARP Books, Scott, Foresman and Company, 1865 Miner Street, Des Plaines, IL 60016. Add $1.75 for shipping and handling.

The Nursing Home Trap. Evaluates home care, residential and nursing-care facilities, nursing home insurance; also looks at Medicare, Medicaid and other benefit programs. Lists caregiver support groups and state and national home-care organizations and associations. Available in book stores or from NOLO Press, 950 parker St, Berkeley, CA 94710. Send check or money order for $16.95 plus $3 shipping. For credit card orders ☏ (800) 992 -6656 (in California, (800) 445-6656.

The following are available free or at reasonable cost from the Alzheimer's Association:

Lincoln, Elizabeth. *Choosing a Nursing Home for the Person with Intellectual Loss*. The Burke Rehabilitation Center. $1.70.

Mace, Nancy L. & Gwyther, Lisa P. *Selecting A Nursing Home With A Dedicated Dementia Care Unit*. $0.80.

The following free literature from the American Association of Retired Persons can be ordered by sending title and stock number to: AARP Fulfillment Section at 1909 K Street, NW, Washington, D.C. 20049:

Nursing Home Life: A Guide for Residents and Families.

The Nursing Home Handbook. $9.95 (AARP members $6.95). To order, write: AARP Books, Scott, Foresman and Company, 1865 Miner Street, Des Plaines, IL 60016. Add $1.75 for shipping and handling.

RESPITE CARE

A Home Away From Home: Consumer Information on Board and Care Homes. #D12446. Send title and stock number to: AARP Fulfillment Section at 1909 K Street, NW, Washington, D.C. 20049.

STRESS, ANXIETY, AND DEPRESSION

Books and Articles:

Beck, Aaron T. *Anxiety Disorders and Phobias: A Cognitive Perspective*. Basic Books.

Beck, Aaron T. *Cognitive Therapy of Depression*. Guilford Press.

Beck, Aaron T. *Cognitive Therapy and The Emotional Disorders*. New American Library.

Benson, Herbert and Miriam Klipper. *The Relaxation Response*. Avon.

Caring For The Caregiver. Free from the Alzheimer's Association.

Carrington, Patricia. *Releasing: The New Behavioral Science Method for Dealing With Pressure Situations*. W. Morrow.

Choosing the Right Therapist for You. Send SASE to American Psychological Association, 750 First St. N.E., Ste 4000, Washington, DC 20002.

Ellis, Albert, et. al., *Handbook of Rational-Emotive Therapy*. Springer Publishing Co.

Hauck, Paul A. *Overcoming Depression*. New York: Institute for Rational-Emotive Therapy. $9.95 ☏ (800) 323-IRET (New York: (212) 535-0822).

Oliver, Rose and Bock, Frances. *Coping With Alzheimer's: A Caregiver's Emotional Survival Guide*. Wilshire Book Company.

If You're Over 65 and Feeling Depressed. Send SASE to: Consumer Information Center, Item 597W, Pueblo, Colo. 81009.

Justice, Blair. *Who Gets Sick*. Jeremy Tarcher.

Standing By You: Family Support Groups. Free from the Alzheimer's Association.

Grandpa Doesn't Know It's Me, by Donna Guthrie. (for children) Human Sciences Press, 1986. ($5.95.)

Tapes:

Tapes like the following are in your local library and video stores:

Beck, Aaron T. *Rational Thinking*.

Beck, Aaron T. *Understanding Anxiety*.

Depression and *Coping with Growing Older*. National Mental Health Association, Information Center, 1021 Prince St., Alexandria, VA 22314-2971. Send SASE for free copy.

Gibson, Dan. *Solitudes: Harmony* (soothing sounds of nature). Hazelden Publishing & Educational Services, 15251 Pleasant

Valley Road, PO Box 176, Center City, MN 55012 ☏ (800) 328-9000, (612) 257-4010 outside the U.S. & Canada.

Goleman, Daniel. *Deep Relaxation.*

Lazarus, Arnold. *Learning to Relax.* New York: Institute for Rational-Emotive Therapy. $9.95 ☏ (800) 323-IRET (New York: (212) 535-0822).

Lehrer, Paul M. *Progressive Relaxation Training.*

Murphy, Cecil. *Day to Day Spiritual Help When Someone You Love Has Alzheimer's.* The Westminster Press.

Rappaport, Alan R. *Relaxation Procedures.*

Stress Management: Coping With Stress. New York: Institute for Rational-Emotive Therapy. $9.95 ☏ (800) 323-IRET (New York: (212) 535-0822).

INDEX